The Pill

John Guillebaud is a consultant gynaecologist at the United Elizabeth Garrett Anderson Hospital and Hospital for Women Soho, in Euston Road, London, and Medical Director of the Margaret Pyke Centre for Study and Training in Family Planning. The Centre was opened by the Duke of Edinburgh in 1969 as a memorial to one of the British pioneers of the family planning movement. It is within the National Health Service, and with about 45,000 annual attendances is the largest fertility centre in Europe. Fertility problems are quite different for different people: thus many couples come to the Centre to avoid an unplanned pregnancy, but others need help in order to start a family. Hundreds of medical students, doctors, and nurses are trained each year at the Centre, and new methods of birth control are investigated with the help of the Margaret Pyke Memorial Trust.

His family came to England more than 300 years ago, with the Huguenots, and so Dr Guillebaud retains the French name as it has always been spelled: it is *pronounced* quite simply '*gil-boe*'. He was born in Burundi, Africa, and educated in Uganda, Kenya, and Britain. In 1959, as an undergraduate at Cambridge, he first awoke to the frightening implications for the future of the world of the population 'explosion', and decided then and there that he would arrange to specialize in Family Planning. Soon after qualifying he spent six months as Medical Officer on the Royal Society Expedition to Mato Grosso, Brazil (1967–8). He has travelled to every continent promoting planned parenthood and concern for the environment, always stressing that human needs cannot be met without action on human numbers. He is a member of several expert committees in the field. His wife Gwyneth is a family planning nurse and they have two sons and one daughter.

John Guillebaud

The Pill

and Other Hormones for Contraception

Fourth Edition

OXFORD UNIVERSITY PRESS

Oxford University Press, Walton Street, Oxford OX2 6DP

Oxford New York Toronto
Delhi Bombay Calcutta Madras Karachi
Petaling Jaya Singapore Hong Kong Tokyo
Nairobi Dar es Salaam Cape Town
Melbourne Auckland

and associated companies in
Berlin Ibadan

First published 1980
Second Edition 1983
Third Edition 1984
Revised reprint 1987
Fourth Edition 1991
Reprinted 1991

British Library Cataloguing in Publication Data
Data available

Library of Congress Cataloging in Publication Data
Guillebaud, John.
The pill / John Guillebaud—4th ed.
p.   cm.
Includes bibliographical references and index.
1. Oral contraceptives.   I. Title.
RG137.5.G84   1991   613.9'432—dc20   91–2457
ISBN 0–19–286126–3

Printed in Great Britain by
Clays Ltd.
Bungay, Suffolk

Preface

to the third edition

Only four years have passed since the first edition. This implies not only that the book is meeting a real need, but also that there continue to be many new developments. The completely rewritten sections include those on cancer, long-term effects of the pill, and 'which pill should be chosen?'. These and a number of smaller, updating changes have been made in the light of the very latest information available in 1984. They are intended to preserve the position of this book as, so far as I know, the most up-to-date and comprehensive handbook on hormonal contraception available anywhere; which in turn explains why it is found on the bookshelves of so many doctors and nurses.

The book could not have been written without the help of many individuals. For reading part or all of the text and making suggestions I am grateful to the following, who are all experts of one kind or another—as researchers, providers, or consumers of the pill: Terry Baker, David Barlow, Toni Belfield, Mary Bollam, Walli Bounds, Peter Bowen-Simpkins, Althea Coates, Heather and Dany Goodman, Meg Goodman, Kathleen Huntington, Clifford Kay, Barbara Law, Audrey Leathard, Jim Mann, Eric McGraw, Alexandra Monks, George Morris, John Newton, Zandria Pauncefort, Walter Prendiville, Maria Pursey, Jan Savage, Pram Senanayake, Susan Sleigh, Gordon Stirrat, and Martin Vessey.

Their comments were supplemented by those of my band of typists, whose patience in typing and retyping drafts was much appreciated: Diana Ager, Margaret Bailón, Eileen Farr, Jeanette Highsted, Irene Jeffery, Julia Kingston-Lee, Nanette Paine, Maxine Stone.

Helpful telephone assistance was provided by Peter Adams, Mark Belsey, Alasdair Breckenridge, Patrick Bye, Max Elstein, Ken Fotherby, and Tom Meade among others. I thank the International Planned Parenthood Federation (IPPF) and Philip

Kestelman in particular for help with the World directory of pill names. The IPPF Wall Chart 'The regulation of fertility' is acknowledged as source material for Figure 23. Figure 2 is reprinted from *International Family Planning Perspectives*, Vol. 5, No. 1 (1979), with permission of the Alan Guttmacher Institute.

My publishers have been most understanding, and I am particularly grateful to Adam Sisman, Hilary Dickinson, Nicola Bion, Angus Phillips, Hilary Feldman, and Peter Clifford for their editorial assistance.

The wisdom in this book comes from many sources. Not all can be mentioned, but all are thanked; and the author must be held responsible for any errors which remain.

Reviewers of the first edition made somewhat contradictory comments: some said that the book would be frightening, some that it displayed a 'pro-pill' bias. Perhaps this suggests that the balance was roughly right. I have been guided throughout by two principles: accuracy about what is known, and honesty about what is still unknown. I deny any conscious bias that would lead to the rejection or watering down of unpalatable facts, of which there are plenty in this book. In making decisions about oral contraception, all the relevant facts must be considered: the benefits as well as the risks of the pill, the risks avoided by taking it (chiefly those of pregnancy), and the risks of the available alternatives. If you read Chapter 6 'The pill in perspective' with an open mind in context with the other chapters, I think you will find that the facts speak for themselves: the pill *is* an appropriate choice for many women— but certainly not for all. A complete consideration of the facts can hardly fail to make anyone pro the pill, at least at their request for those I have called 'the safer women'—primarily healthy young women who do not smoke cigarettes. But there are other methods available even for them.

Never forget that you have a choice.

Some readers will disagree with my opinions or policies, and this is fine. There is still so much we do not yet know, experts disagree about how much weight to give to the facts that are known, and new facts may well emerge after publication. So much depends on people's attitudes, life-styles, and religious beliefs. Indeed, these issues warrant books of their own, and discussion of them and of other important topics has had to be brief.

Though one day there may be a usable male pill (see Chapter 9), I cannot, of course, write as a consumer . . . just as an understanding prescriber. Indeed, although the book is intended primarily for women considering or already taking the pill, I have been pleased to learn how many men have found it helpful.

Finally, I thank my parents for much guidance and practical help. And to my wife Gwyneth I owe an incalculable debt. Her advice and constructive criticism have been derived from practical experience, both as a family planning nurse and as a woman, a wife, and the mother of our three energetic children.

John Guillebaud, MA, FRCSE, FRCOG

Medical Director
Margaret Pyke Centre for Study and
Training in Family Planning

Opinions on oral contraception vary—from those expressed by the Pill Victims' Action Group to those of many thousands of women who find it an excellent method of birth control. This book is based on evidence available at the time of writing.

Preface

to the fourth edition

This actually represents the fifth version of the book in ten years. Updating changes have been necessary on the majority of pages. AIDS has loomed as a completely new problem, new progestogens have become established, and the sections on 'missed pills' and cancer have been completely rewritten.

In addition to those mentioned in the preface to the third edition, I should like to acknowledge the help of all my colleagues at the Margaret Pyke Centre, including Suzy Hatwell (Sister in Charge), Sister Maddy Ward, Sister Sarah Raynor, and Pat Sullivan (Administrator). Ali Kubba, until recently my Deputy at the Centre, helped by acting as a sounding-board for various ideas, and especially by treating my patients at the Centre and Hospital during my inevitable absences. Lady Jean Medawar, the Director of The Margaret Pyke Memorial Trust, has been and continues to be enormously supportive of all our work at the Centre, and the Trust supplied the word processor on which my son Jonathan retyped the whole book. Dr Anne Szarewski read through the whole revised third edition and made numerous specific suggestions for improvements.

John Guillebaud

Contents

List of figures   x

List of tables   xi

How to use this book   1

Introduction   3

1. **Sex and contraception: yesterday, today, and everywhere**   7

2. **The pill: how does it work?**   32

3. **The pill: how do I take it?**   52

4. **The pill: will it make me ill? Diseases of the circulation**   85

5. **Other effects of the pill**   108

6. **The pill in perspective**   157

7. **Who for the pill, and which pill for you?**   171

8. **The progestogen-only pill (mini-pill)**   207

9. **The future of family planning: and what became of the male pill?**   226

10. **All things considered: shall I take the pill?**   250

100 questions everyone asks about the pill   261

Postscript   280

Glossary   283

Further reading   290

Useful addresses   295

World directory of pill names   301

Index   307

List of figures

1.	Number of deaths per year for 100,000 people at risk	6
2.	The pill	7
3.	What changes birth rates?	15
4.	How birth control methods are used by women in Great Britain	21
5.	The female reproductive system: control of the menstrual cycle	33
6.	Close-up of ovary to show growth of follicles and formation of corpus luteum after egg-release	35
7.	(a) The menstrual cycle (b) Early pregnancy	36
8.	How the combined pill prevents pregnancy	45
9.	The pill cycle (21-day system)	48
10.	Diary card—first day start of the pill	56
11a.	The pill cycle (21-day system)	60
11b.	What to do when pills are taken late or missed altogether	61
12.	What to do in the event of a stomach upset	68
13.	Influence of pill-use, smoking, and age on overall death rates due to diseases of the circulation	106
14.	Chance of being diagnosed with breast cancer, in young women aged 35 or less	140
15.	Cancer and the pill: a balance	146
16.	The effect of the pill on the rate of occurrence of some selected conditions	160
17.	Pill ladders	190
18.	Two possible methods for short-term postponement of withdrawal bleeding (WTB) by women using phasic pills	195
19.	Which pill?	198
20.	Which pill? Bleeding patterns	200
21.	What to do if progestogen-only pills are taken late or a stomach upset occurs	212
22.	The progestogen-only contraceptive vaginal ring	223
23.	The stages of reproduction	230
24.	An immune method: anti-hCG antibodies stop early pregnancy from maintaining corpus luteum	238

List of tables

1. Percentage contraceptive use in each age-group of British women   22
2. How combined pills prevent pregnancy   46
3. Drugs which are suspected of interfering with the pill, to cause 'breakthrough' bleeding and increased risk of pregnancy   70
4. Some changes in body chemistry   88
5. Reduction in hormone dose given since combined pills were first introduced   154
6. Blood pressure according to dose of progestogen   155
7. Side-effects of the combined pill   158
8. How to have a (very low) 1 in 1 million risk of dying   166
9. Ultra-low-dose combined pills with less than 50 mcg of oestrogen available in the UK   186
10. 'Ordinary' low-dose combined pills—all containing 50 mcg of oestrogen—available in the UK   188
11. How progestogen-only pills prevent pregnancy   208
12. Brands of progestogen-only pills available in Britain   221
13. Features of the ideal contraceptive   226
14. The main recommended and widely available methods of birth control   251
15. The seven contraceptive ages of woman   257

How to use this book

The Pill can be read straight through, or dipped into as a reference book. You may well prefer to skip those sections marked with an asterisk (*) which are mainly for those who are interested in the finer details. But however you read it, be sure to include Chapter 6 which may help you to see 'the pill in perspective'.

Another possibility is to look first at the section '100 questions everyone asks about the pill' (page 261). The brief answer there may be all you need: but if you want a more detailed account the pages to read are also given.

Unless otherwise stated the word 'pill' on its own means the ordinary combined pill containing two hormones, an oestrogen and a progestogen, as explained in Chapter 2.

You, your doctor, and the pill

Doctors who still have a kind of 'God complex' and expect all their decisions to be taken on trust, with no discussion, will not like this book. I hope that there will be few such or at least that they refrain from telling people what method of family planning they should use. If the pill is the method in question, in most countries doctors and nurses do the advising and the supplying, but they should not do the *deciding: that is your right*.

None the less, even the most human and communicative doctors are unlikely to appreciate being told that you read in this or any other book what they should do next in your case! Make allowances for the fact that your clinic or family doctor has much experience, and may have very good reasons for disagreeing with something suggested here. The golden rule is, if you are ever in doubt about any aspect of pill-use, make sure that you talk things over with someone you trust, who knows the answers.

One problem shared by all doctors is lack of time. So I think most will be delighted if you are so well informed about the pill having read this book, that by the time you come to their surgery or clinic you only have one or two points left to clear up.

And if the pill is not for you ...

If the pill does not suit you, or if for some reason you must avoid or give up the pill, remember the choice is not between the pill and nothing; the *coil* (intra-uterine device: IUD), the *cap* (or diaphragm), and the *sheath* (condom) can all provide very effective reversible contraception. The last of these has become especially relevant since earlier editions of this book, due to the new need to consider the vital matter of protection against the virus causing AIDS. Indeed in the waiting-room of the Margaret Pyke Centre we have a large easel bearing a notice reminding all present that '*we also supply condoms*'— *which may need to be used as well, whatever your method of birth control.* See pages 23–8 for more about sexually transmitted diseases.

Do not forget that there are also important hormone options which are not 'the pill', especially the *progestogen-only pill* (POP), which used to be called the mini-pill, and *injectables*— see Chapters 8 and 9 for more details. And Chapter 10 gives a brief account of the other methods, including sterilization.

It is important to choose carefully, as the wrong choice can lead to problems; not least an unwanted pregnancy, either by using an inefficient method, or by using a better method inefficiently. The main reason why contraception seems such an unavoidable bore, or rather why it is often actually avoided, is that all our present reversible methods are tried and found wanting in some way. They either have side-effects, or are a nuisance and interfere with love-making. So Chapter 9 deals with attempts to produce better methods for the future.

Introduction

by Gwyneth Guillebaud, RGN, ONC, FPA Cert.

Every day over 70 million women reach out for a pill packet and swallow a tiny tablet which alters the course of their lives. Approaching 200 million have done so at some time. And millions more will do so.

What that means to you—whether you are taking the pill yourself, have at some time taken it, or are thinking of doing so, whether you love someone who is taking it, or are in some other way involved or interested in oral contraceptives—what it means to all of us in fact is what this book is about.

The pill, very largely developed by men, produced by men, marketed by men, prescribed by men (written about by men!), and also undoubtedly of benefit to men, is taken by women. Should we as women be thankful? Thirty years ago when the pill became available, first in America, then elsewhere, that question would have been very much easier to answer. It seemed that at last there was an answer to the prayer of so many couples through the ages—contraception without complication. Simple and safe. The publicity was enormous, expectations were high.

What now, after three decades? *Should* we be thankful? Many of us, feminists and non-feminists alike, who have come to see control of fertility as a necessity, a right, and a freedom, would now like to respond by asking further questions. Is the price for this freedom too high? Does taking the pill mean taking control or being controlled? Moreover, who has gained the freedom? Has the pill liberated men more than women? It is hard to deny that many men have come to *assume* that women will take it. Why won't they take their own share of responsibility?

The pill has not lived up to all expectations, and women have become understandably cautious. There have been numerous press articles on the risks of the pill, and although many were unjustifiably scary, others were accurate. They have given some cause to question the medical safety of the pill method.

But if that is the case, why do so many women continue to reach regularly for the pill packet? There are several good reasons. Being an ostrich is not one of them. What is needed is a balance of healthy caution and practical common sense. The best reason for taking the pill is that it works. Whatever else experience has shown, it has proved that oral contraception is easy and effective. Secondly, once stripped of sensationalism, the weight of informed opinion is that the risks relate to a very small number of women. Over the years it has become much easier to single out those who are at particular risk and the doses used in current pills are much reduced and believed to be correspondingly safer.

Whatever the range of opinions about the pill, many women in modern society consider it a necessity. At an everyday and practical level, it has relieved millions of women from the constant fear of unwanted pregnancy. For all those who do experience side-effects, there are many who take it without problems and with great relief that a major aspect of their lives is no longer a source of stress. Our grandmothers were less fortunate.

Yet the introduction to the first edition of *The Pill* mentioned a British survey which revealed that of 1,000 women using the pill, one in three felt her health was being damaged and not properly monitored.

I can readily sympathize with those women—writing as a woman, with a woman's concerns about my body and the impact on it of contraception, and particularly the pill. As a contraceptive user, I have tried practically all the recommended reversible methods with a record of success and occasional failure, of overall satisfaction, but also of having to live with some side-effects.

To reject all contraception or use very unsafe methods, as some couples do, simply because the ideal method does not exist, is to put the clock right back. That is not freedom. We should avoid having unrealistic expectations. Almost nothing in life is completely safe and free of all health risks. Like every drug that has ever been devised, the pill can cause side-effects. And you are continually being reminded that it might do you harm by the tablet that you swallow each day. However, when I took it I reminded myself that the betting odds were overwhelmingly in my favour.

Although every one of our current methods of family planning has one snag or another, I have proved like many other women that it is possible to find an acceptable method for every stage of our life. Of course I am lucky, having a husband who is particularly well informed! But even more important than the information is a good relationship, the freedom to discuss one's feelings and fears. The eventual decision should ideally be a joint one.

Nevertheless if the method is one to be used by a woman, then the woman should make the final decision. The weight of medical opinion believes that for many women the known advantages of the pill far outweigh any possible risks. But it is for the individual woman to decide whether she can be confident it is really right for her—whatever a doctor, or family planning nurse, or anyone else may say. She must weigh up many considerations: how big a risk of pregnancy might be accepted, how easy the method is, the likelihood and nature of side-effects, the acceptability of other alternatives, and personal preferences. We live our lives and base our decisions on what we know, and the best and right decisions are those for which we feel we have taken responsibility.

That is why accurate knowledge is essential. The introduction to the first edition described this book as 'a handbook for the owner/driver of a healthy pill-taking body'. That is still the approach.

The facts as far as they are known are here. They may confirm your doubts about the pill. They may equally give you new confidence in it. It is up to you now to make the decisions.

G. M. G.

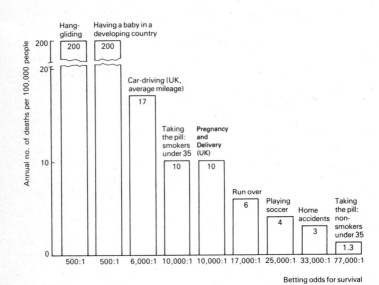

Fig. 1 Number of deaths per year for 100,000 people at risk

Notes: The implications of this figure are discussed on pages 165–7. The risks of pill-taking for smokers or non-smokers concern circulatory disease, and relate to older pills containing at least 50 mcg oestrogen. Cancer is not in the reckoning since, as explained on pages 138–46, the benefits of the pill in *cancer protection* are believed more or less to cancel out the possible adverse effects.

The risks of pregnancy and delivery in all countries are much higher than pill-taking for non-smokers under 35. This statistic is not given to scare UK women about having a baby, since 10,000 to 1 in your favour represents pretty good odds. The point is the pill is even safer (and *prevents* pregnancy).

PS Since the last edition, research now shows that modern pills containing less than 50 mcg of oestrogen are safer even than the figure suggests. Indeed an adverse effect of pill-taking cannot now be detected unless women *also* smoke (see page 105).

6 Sex and contraception

I

···

Sex and contraception yesterday, today, and everywhere

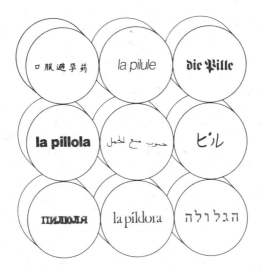

Fig. 2

The pill has spread far and wide throughout the world. It is no exaggeration to say that it has changed the course of recent history: not so much directly as indirectly by subtle changes in people's thinking, attitudes, and behaviour.

This first chapter covers a few subjects which are connected with or affected by the pill. They all deserve a mention, indeed each could have had a whole book devoted to it. If your appetite is whetted see Further reading (page 290).

Human fertility and the history of contraception

We break no records in the animal kingdom, but we are a remarkably fertile species. Doctors and others who work in family planning rapidly develop a great respect for human sperm! First seen under the microscope 300 years ago, they were initially thought to be 'parasites'. It was not until the 1840s that it was realized that they were crucial to the whole process of fertilization and the creation of a new individual. Millions of them are released at every act of intercourse when the man reaches climax. If each sperm in a normal man's ejaculate were able to find an egg the resulting number of pregnancies would be over 300 million, enough to populate the whole of North America! They come off the 'production line' at his testicles at the rate of 1,000 sperm a second, night and day until old age. Every single one of them has its own 'outboard motor' and knows exactly where it wants to go.

Unless something is done to stop them, the sperm get into the uterus (womb) within a minute or so of being deposited in the woman's vagina. If she has a climax (an orgasm), it seems that they may actually be sucked into the uterus; however, avoidance of a climax most certainly does *not* protect the woman from pregnancy. Although they will die in a very short time in the vagina, once they get into the uterus they have remarkable powers of survival. They like it there: it has often been written that 'sperm might fertilize an egg for three or four days' . . . Modern research suggests that that is the *average* sperm's survival: with 300 million plus arriving what matters is the survival of the 'lunatic fringe'! This can be six or even (rarely) seven days. These facts explain many unplanned pregnancies which occur after love-making at a time that many people think is safe, around the end of a woman's period. When she later produces her egg she may conceive as a result of that single act of unprotected intercourse as much as a *week* earlier. The risk is even greater if like most women she sometimes has cycles which are shorter than the average of 28 days, meaning that her egg comes earlier than the usual, which is day 14 (page 34). Hence for many women it is wrong to claim that this early phase of the cycle is part of the 'safe period' at all. It is not the time to make love without precautions, unless you want or can accept a baby. See page 240 for more about research to improve the effectiveness of 'natural family planning'.

As far as nature is concerned, intercourse is designed to produce babies and ensure the survival of the species. Sex is also exciting and pleasurable, and especially so between two people who really love and care for each other. This helps to ensure that pregnancies do happen, and that the babies will survive because food and shelter are provided by their parents (see page 30). But if nature had its way each fertile woman could have a baby every year or two from the age of about 15 to over 40. For a long time past this has seemed a bit too much of a good thing.

It is not surprising therefore that methods of preventing pregnancy have been looked for and often practised. Right from the start in many societies they appear to have been frowned on. One of the main reasons was the fact that a high birth rate was essential for survival of the species. Both infant and adult mortality were extremely high and large numbers of children had to be born simply to ensure that each generation replaced itself. Medical advances have now controlled many of the killing diseases of the past, so that in the twentieth century we are faced with the quite different problem of a population explosion. But at various times in the last three or four thousand years it has been said that family planning even within marriage is dangerous, sinful, antisocial, a threat to posterity, a form of witchcraft . . . Doctors have been as confused as anyone. Speaking to the British Medical Association in 1878, a Dr Routh said that 'sexual fraudulency' (his name for contraception) using the sheath or female barriers or spermicides might cause in one or other sex a whole range of diseases. These included cancer, mania leading to suicide, general nervous prostration, mental decay, loss of memory, and intense cardiac palpitations.

Nevertheless, the search for birth control methods continued. The earliest workers were highly unscientific and the methods they came up with were frequently useless, often uncomfortable, and sometimes ridiculous. In 1850 BC the Petri Papyrus from Egypt described the use of crocodile dung made into a paste and put into the vagina, or alternatively, a mixture whose chief ingredient was honey. Other nasty brews which could in fact have been effective as barriers, and sometimes also because of their sperm-killing effects, included cabbage, pitch, ox gall, and elephant dung, to be used 'alone or in combination'. This was favoured by one Rhazes who died in about AD 923. A later Arab report suggested the use of the right testicle of a wolf wrapped in oil-soaked wool! There is not much point in trying to list all the confused ideas. But it is interesting that some of the myths which some people still believe today have a very long history. Soranos, who wrote during the second century AD, suggested that the woman should 'hold back' (i.e. avoid having an orgasm) to prevent semen entering her uterus. She should then get up, sneeze, and drink something cold. Rhazes said something similar and added that she should jump backwards seven or nine times in order to dislodge the semen.

However, again from the earliest times, the ideal method was felt to be an *oral* contraceptive, which would avoid the need for doing something artificial and messy at the time of intercourse itself. In ancient China women were advised to swallow twenty-four live tadpoles in the early spring and they would then have five years free of conception. Albert the Great in the Middle Ages suggested bees should be eaten rather than tadpoles . . . talk about side-effects of oral contraception! . . . North African tribes once drank a gunpowder solution made with the foam gathered from sweating flanks of their camels. None of these methods is likely actually to have worked, and some such as those based on arsenic or strychnine probably saw off more women than sperm!

However, there were various potions based on plants; the Greek herbals of the first few centuries AD mentioned many. Anthropologists have accumulated from the folklore of primitive peoples all over the world the names of literally hundreds of plants which are believed to prevent or interrupt pregnancy. They have been made up into a variety of concoctions, often referred to as bush teas, and it is possible that a very few may really have had the desired effect. Some of the plants have been shown to contain oestrogens and so could have worked in the same sort of way as the pill (see Chapter 2). Others may have worked through alkaloids and similar substances not yet identified, either to stop fertilization or to cause abortion by contractions of the uterus. Indeed, research workers believe that somewhere in the rain forests of the world, in among the mumbo-jumbo, there may be a plant medicine in use from time immemorial which could provide the clue to a new and safe oral contraceptive. Another reason why it is such a tragedy to allow 100 acres of tropical rain forest to be destroyed per minute (see below)! For some years the World Health Organization had a Task Force looking into indigenous plant products. Although its work did not result directly in any new drugs, the most promising leads are still being followed up in various Centres.

The *Dioscorea* plant is a wild yam vine which clings to trees in the mountains of southern Mexico. Its coal-black roots used to be harvested by the Mexican Indians for the production of the substance diosgenin, which was formerly the source of most of the hormones required for making pills. Because of a world shortage of these yams, aggravated by the fact that they have never been successfully cultivated, alternative raw materials for making the hormones are now used. (The modern history of the development of oral contraception for women is described in the next chapter.)

Going back to the Ancients, oral contraception for the male was not entirely neglected. For instance, a man called Aetios, who wrote in the sixth century AD, recommended the burned testicles of the mule, drunk with a decoction of willow. The mule may well have been chosen because it is of course a sterile animal. In Chapter 9 I shall be considering research to produce rather more effective oral contraceptives for men.

The pill and the world scene

We have fought disease, we are eliminating malaria . . . and the age of expectancy of life has gone up, and we have reduced child mortality. But believe me, . . . all this is like writing in the sand. You write in the sand and the tide of population comes in and wipes out all that is written.

M. C. Chagla, High Commissioner for India, 1963: speaking at an FPA symposium at Church House, Westminster.

In recent years the birth rate in Western industrialized countries has fallen dramatically. The situation in much of the rest of the world is very different. It used to be said: 'There is one born every second.' The truth is much nearer five per second. In round terms, based on the latest (1990) figures of the Population Reference Bureau, Washington DC, every 10 seconds 46 people are born on to this planet of ours. In the same time, 17 adults or children die. The difference means that 29 extra individuals have to be accommodated every 10 seconds, or about 1,000 average jumbo jet flights every day, a million newcomers every four days. World population will certainly double and could easily treble before stability is achieved.

Two-thirds of planet earth is ocean and much of the remainder is mountain or desert. It has taken perhaps 10,000 years since agriculture was first practised for world population to reach its present total of 5,400 million. If the same number again are to arrive by 2150 (a conservative estimate), and we are going to meet their most basic needs even as *badly* as we do for our present world, then we are going to have to double *everything*. For every house in the world we will need another house; for every school another school; for every hospital another hospital. Another world's worth of people will require at least as much again of food and clothing as is available now to the world of the early 1990s. A pretty daunting prospect: especially when you add three further facts.

First, there is no humane way that at least one further doubling can be avoided. The parents of all these new people are already born. Of the world's population 33 per cent is under the age of 15 and in many developing countries the figure is 40–50 per cent. If by some miracle Mr and Mrs World Citizen had on average only the number of children required for replacement (a little over two), starting tomorrow, the population of the whole world would still not stabilize until there were about 10,000 million people.

Second, birth rates, although falling in most countries in the developing world, are in fact a very long way above the replacement level. For this reason we may have to contemplate catering for three worlds of the present size. Continuing imbalance between birth rates and death rates is not an option:

if humanity fails to balance the numbers by better birth planning, Nature's most unwelcome solution will occur instead on a gigantic scale: i.e. a massive increase in the number of deaths which could be due to famine, epidemics, or of course wars.

Third, and most important, two-thirds of the people in the world even now lack a bare minimum of the requirements for reasonable health and comfort. Suppose the impossible were achieved and all the requirements of the world were doubled as just described. Unless the present unjust and unequal distribution of the world's wealth—itself a great wrong—were also put right at each level of need, the *percentage* of deprived people would remain unchanged. With a doubling of world numbers that would mean *twice as many* destitute as there are now.

The complex and interrelated environmental problems facing the world are discussed in many books (e.g. *Only One Earth*—see Further reading). It is clear that we must cease being such an arrogant species, forever treating this beautiful but vulnerable planet as an inexhaustible milch cow (for resources) and as a bottomless cess-pit (for pollution). But much of the damage is not wilful, it comes from there being too many of us. *How can we expect to check pollution and resource consumption without stabilizing the number of polluters and resource consumers?* Every two seconds more than three acres of tropical rain forest are destroyed. The greenhouse effect, the destruction of the ozone layer, threatened wildlife with over a million species likely to be extinct by the year 2000, energy shortages, Gulf conflicts, terrorism: can you think of an important world problem which is not worsened by the number of humans? Floods in Bangladesh are caused by soil-erosion from too many tree-cutters in Nepal; and then more people drown each flood as ever more are forced by population pressure to live in areas which everyone knows are subject to inundation . . .

Nearer to home, the endangered species of Britain are mainly threatened by destruction of their habitats—by humans. This would be *far less if the UK had not previously had its own population explosion*. With more affluence, more and more people are able to have the car and the house and garden in the country they have always wanted, the traffic jams proliferate and the environment deteriorates. What a 'green and pleasant land' would be ours if we had stabilized at the 20 million which John Stuart Mill considered already sufficient 150 years ago. Truly, *whatever your cause it is a lost cause unless we tackle population*.

Roughly speaking, every new birth in 'over-developed' countries like Britain and America will lead during the lifetime of that person to something between 30 and 40 times more impact on the environment than a new arrival in a poor country like, say, Uganda. Each of us in the rich countries behaves like one cog in a vast machine which eats up raw materials of all kinds at one end, and spews out rubbish at the other. 'Over-population' is certainly not just a problem for the poor countries as we may like to think.

Yet population is the 'Cinderella' of both the Green movement and of development efforts. It is seen as a 'hot potato' and so as a CONSTANT to which we must always adapt: rather than the root cause of much of the misery to come, and one we could actually tackle.

But it is not by any means just a (human) numbers game. The solution is not solely to stabilize or reduce population. Many other changes are necessary including, a lot of people would believe, substantially more effective help for the less developed countries by the rich ones; and rejection of the often wasteful philosophy that 'Biggest is best'. Much better slogans are: 'Small is beautiful' and 'Enough is enough'—see books with these titles (page 293).

'The rich get richer and the poor get children'

The toll of human misery caused by excessive fertility is great. Every year 500,000 maternal deaths occur due to pregnancy (one every minute), all but 6,000 in the Third World. Fifteen million children die each year (one every 2 seconds) before the age of 5, partly from malnutrition. And annually there are something between 30 and 40 million induced abortions, at least half of them illegal and causing much death and injury, or permanent infertility. Surveys have repeatedly shown that many of the pregnancies that result in so many deaths of mothers and babies were unwanted in the first place. So family planning can and should reduce this ghastly death toll, not to mention the emotional trauma for all the families involved.

Many obstacles

Why, with a few exceptions, are most of the developing countries still so far from stabilizing their population numbers? Early efforts to provide voluntary family planning in the Third World failed on two counts. They failed to appreciate, according to a saying from the Far East, that 'every mouth has got two hands'. For the individual family unit in rural poverty, the hands (the work a child can do for the family) seem more important than the mouth. Secondly, family planning may seem irrelevant when there is a high infant mortality rate. It is now at least understood, though far too little practised, that the best way to achieve an effective voluntary solution to the population problem is by a fully comprehensive approach (see Figure 3). *'Take care of the people and the population will take care of itself.'*

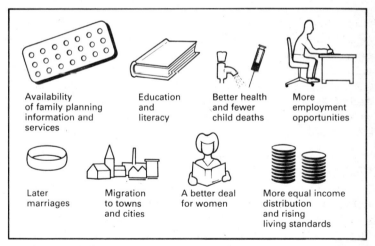

| Availability of family planning information and services | Education and literacy | Better health and fewer child deaths | More employment opportunities |
| Later marriages | Migration to towns and cities | A better deal for women | More equal income distribution and rising living standards |

Fig. 3 What changes birth rates?

Source: The Shape of Things to Come, Population Concern.

But it is a misinterpretation of this true saying to declare that family planning is therefore unimportant. In large areas of the world the basic tools for the family planning job are just not available. *'Population will take care of itself'* only when *'taking care of the people'* includes all aspects of appropriate development (including education and literacy, improved health, housing, and above all women's rights) as part of a package—but a package which *includes* providing, as a human right, the methods of birth control which people actually want now in the slums and rural areas where people actually live, now.

There are many other obstacles to be overcome, hopefully by education and more responsible programming by the media: wrong priorities in funding (guns before pills); competitive breeding; false teaching and 'flat earthism' among many religious leaders—not only the Pope; male-dominated attitudes with double standards (like the men in Third World cities who say their wives 'might be unfaithful' if not at home having babies, yet themselves regularly go with prostitutes); fatalism; and above all *apathy*.

Apathy partly results because in all countries we just don't see the 'writ large' effects of what we all individually do: we say 'The crowds at the shops today were awful' and forget that we caused the crowds just as much as anyone else did. 'My car is my car: everybody else's car is traffic!' . . . 'The death of one baby, that's a tragedy: the death of millions of babies, that is a statistic' . . . Really? And finally: 'My baby is my baby: everybody else's baby, that's overpopulation.'

And what about perhaps the greatest obstacles of all?—the biological drive of sex and all those millions of sperm.

Voluntary, available, methods
The massive World Fertility Survey found on average almost 50 per cent of married women in the developing world wanted no more children (80 per cent in some countries). But most lacked access to the methods that would enable them to avoid having more. So despite all those obstacles to acceptance of family planning, there already is an enormous perceived need for it, and one which is not being met. Surely, every couple in the world should be able to use contraceptive methods if they really

do so wish—as a human right, let alone for population reasons! Because there are so few doctors, especially in country areas, a committee of international experts has said, 'Whoever normally meets the health needs of the community, whether doctor, nurse, traditional midwife, pharmacist or store-keeper would be an appropriate person to distribute oral contraceptives, supported by adequate information, education and medical back-up services.' This idea of using non-doctors even to distribute the pill is controversial: it should be discussed in the light of the often astronomically high relative risks of unplanned pregnancy in the community concerned (see *The Pill off Prescription*, Further reading). But community-based distribution of the barriers and spermicides is hazard-free and voluntary and should be happening routinely everywhere now.

What can I do?
Faced with all this opposition, it is easy to 'cop-out' since 'anything I could do would be but a drop in the ocean' . . . forgetting that 'the ocean is made up of drops'. Population Concern, the Margaret Pyke Memorial Trust, the Conservation Trust, Marie Stopes International, and the World Wide Fund for Nature are key organizations worthy of support since they are prepared to grasp the population nettle. They are concerned to preserve at least a half-way decent world for all the world's children to inherit as well as for other species sharing the planet (see Useful addresses, pages 296, 300, for Britain).

Oxfam on the other hand, like most Development agencies, badly need to come up to date: maybe, dear reader, you can help to apply some polite pressure in this area? Oxfam seem to have forgotten their own slogan of some years ago, 'Unborn children don't starve.' Their programmes do sometimes include family planning, but they fail to give it the *high profile* it deserves. Oxfam teaches us, rightly, to 'love our neighbour' *overseas*. But they need also to show much more concern for our *future* neighbours—who can best be helped by not being too numerous (i.e. by family planning).

Nothing I have just said is particularly new and the facts must be known to the politicians and rulers of most countries of the world. Yet there is far too much windy rhetoric and not enough appropriate action. Will future generations condemn this one for missing the last opportunity to enable them to inherit a habitable world? The stakes are high and the 1990s are crucial, since only a few years' delay in achieving near-universal availability of voluntary family planning in the Third World during this decade means that we will have to cater for 15,000 million (two extra worlds) rather than that unavoidable 10,000 million in the next century. And if all the world's inhabitants were able to live the affluent life-styles to which all aspire, the planet could only sustain a maximum of about 2,000 million people . . . less than half of the number already here. *Human needs cannot be met without tackling human numbers.*

A final thought: it has been said, and it is probably true, that

> *more babies are prevented worldwide by breast-feeding than by all the world's family planning programmes put together.*

This does not contradict the well-known fact that if individual couples rely solely on breast-feeding for family planning, they are liable to be let down. (To have a really good contraceptive effect, breast-feeding must be intensive, as practised traditionally in many developing countries: the baby must receive no supplementary feeds. See page 240.) What this statement means is that if almost all women in a community do breast-feed their children, their overall fertility is reduced. Certainly, if breast-feeding becomes infrequent—a most unwelcome trend in most areas—the interval between children is much shorter (with, in fact, a doubling of the infant mortality rate if it becomes less than two years).

The other thing the statement shows, of course, is how *terrifyingly inadequate* are all the world's family planning programmes put together!

The pill and women's role in society

> The pill has fallen from its pedestal to take its place among the other contraceptives, each with flaws and assets . . . [But] without the advent of the pill and women's response to the freedom it *promised*, our present age would clearly be very different, and so would our vision of the future.
>
> Susan Scrimshaw, *Family Planning Perspectives*, 1982

In some countries, mostly but not exclusively less developed, the status of women has to be improved before much headway can be made in introducing the idea of family limitation by any methods. But it is also true that in many other societies the pill, above all other methods of family planning, has helped to bring about major changes in the role of women. This is because, for the first time, women have the option to decide how many children to have, when to have them, and whether to have them at all. Now they no longer necessarily have to be constantly child-bearing and child-rearing. Marriage and the first child can be and are delayed (this can be overdone, however, see page 126). Women are free to proceed to higher education and to pursue independent careers far more than in the past. So it is probably no coincidence that the pill has been widely available for the last 25 years in most Western countries, and over the same period movements for women's rights and equal opportunities have become more effective. There is still a long way to go, however: would the world tolerate one person dying every minute from childbirth if men had babies? Many job and other opportunities in all countries without exception are simply not available to women.

Some women still prefer their main role in life to be that of wife and mother. They should not feel inferior for not aspiring to be engineers or Prime Ministers. Neither should the aspiring engineers feel bad for not opting for parenthood. The right to choose is the main thing and this exists far more now than in the days before the pill.

Nature was very unkind in placing so very many of the problems connected with having babies on the one sex. Problems with the sexual apparatus of women can happen at any time, particularly at puberty and through the fertile years (pre-menstrual tension, painful or heavy periods, and all the troubles of child-bearing), at the menopause, and even in old age. Men, on the other hand, get off virtually scot-free, with almost nothing to worry about apart from a bit of prostate trouble and that usually not until they are past the age of 70. The pill has helped to even out this imbalance between the sexes: not only by its obvious effect in reducing the frequency and hence the risks of child-bearing, but also because it so commonly improves the menstrual cycle. But the pill for women also has many drawbacks, of course. So even more welcome will be the day when a male pill is available, so that men can take more of a share in the whole business of family planning (see Chapter 9).

Usage of the pill in the world—and in the United Kingdom

The proportion of pill-users in each country of the world varies enormously, from less than 1 per cent of women of child-bearing age to around 40 per cent (or even 70 per cent in selected groups of younger women). Usage in most of the less developed countries is relatively low for the reasons given earlier. But even in countries without those obstacles, the proportion of women using the pill can be low, depending on the alternatives available, and sometimes for religious reasons (as in Italy or Ireland) or for reasons of medico-politics (Japan).

In spite of many worrying newspaper articles, the United Kingdom is an example of a country where the pill continues to be very commonly used—as shown in Table 1 and Figure 4. Among sexually active women aged 16 to 29 surveyed by the Royal College of General Practitioners in 1985 only 5 per cent had never taken it at all! Even in 1990 there still seem to be around three million current users in the UK.

It is a rapidly moving scene: even since Table 1 was compiled the condom has been increasingly chosen by those seeking protection against sexually transmitted diseases, especially AIDS. It is often used *as well as* the pill. What is more, in a 1989 survey for Durex by the Henley Centre around 20 per cent of 5,000 couples interviewed used the sheath as their main method, compared with just 19 per cent using the pill. But in the 18 to 30 age-group the pill remained more popular as the main method (used by 32–8 per cent). Over age 30, sterilization is becoming so popular that, if current trends continue, in a clear majority of couples one or other of the partners will have been sterilized by the time the wife is 35.

In Table 1 it is clear that even today many do not appear to be using a fully effective method of birth control and yet are not trying to become pregnant. We know too from the large and

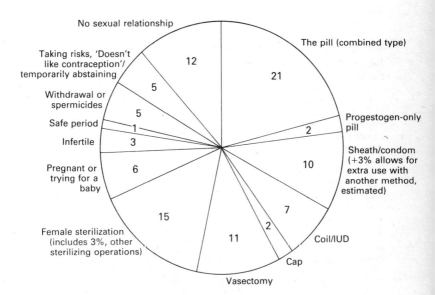

Fig. 4 How birth control methods are used by women in Great Britain. Data from General Household Survey, see Table 1

Note: The percentages shown are out of a total of about 13 million women in the age-group 16–49.

Condom use with/without another method has gone up since the above figures were obtained, to about 20 per cent use as the 'main method' (Henley Centre Study, 1989). This increase is attributed to couples' concern to prevent AIDS.

Table I Percentage contraceptive use in some age-groups of British women

	16–17	20–4	25–9	30–4	40–4	All ages (16–49)
Method of contraception						
Pill	20	55	38	21	4	23
Condom	6	9	13	15	14	13
IUD	1	4	9	11	7	7
Cap	—	2	3	4	2	2
Withdrawal/safe period/ spermicides/other	2	6	7	7	9	6
Sterilization						
Female	—	1	3	10	28	12
Male	—	—	4	15	20	11
TOTAL USERS	27	72	71	79	81	71
Reasons for non-use of contraception						
No sexual relationship	54	13	7	6	6	12
(Temporarily) abstaining to avoid pregnancy	15	4	2	1	1	3
Pregnant	2	6	9	5	0	4
Wanting to conceive	—	3	5	4	1	2
Doesn't like contraception	1	1	2	2	2	2
Post-menopause or sterile after other operation (e.g. hysterectomy)	—	—	1	1	7	4
Possibly infertile	—	—	1	1	2	2
Other (including breast-feeding)	1	1	2	4	3	0
TOTAL NON-USERS	73	28	29	21	19	29

Notes: 1. Figures reported in a UK FPA Factsheet (Feb. 1990), derived from the British General Household Survey. This was published in 1989 from data collected in 1986.
2. Numbers in the columns may add to more than 100 due to rounding and because some women used more than one reversible method.

now increasing number of requests for termination of pregnancy (abortion) that many who say in surveys that they are using a particular method like the sheath actually take risks from time to time ... More of these couples need to know about emergency contraception (see page 78); but they also need to 'get their act together' and use a well-chosen method more consistently.

A similar amount of risk-taking continues today in all the other developed countries. Yet almost no one can plead the excuse of ignorance or of the methods just not being available, as they could in say Burundi or Nepal. We seem not to know how lucky we are!

Unwanted pregnancy

'Most accidents are caused by a human and most humans are caused by an accident.' Thanks to the pill this is less true than it once was. But a high percentage of today's parents did not plan their first, or their latest, arrival. Being pregnant when you do not want to be is a good recipe for guilt feelings and much personal misery, not to mention family rows and money crises. It is not impossible, of course, for an unwanted pregnancy to lead eventually to the birth of a wanted, loved, and well-cared-for child. However, this may well not be the outcome.

And whatever people say, the usual alternative to keeping the baby—abortion—leads to emotional scarring and regret . . .

But I am sure you would not be reading this book if you were not already convinced that children should come by loving choice rather than careless chance.

The pill and sexually transmitted diseases

I considered the 'population explosion' earlier but there is another recent phenomenon, the 'copulation explosion'. If the effects of the former seem a bit remote, those of the latter can be a bit too close for comfort. An increasing number of people nowadays expect more sex more often and with less commitment. Three pretty obvious statements can be made about this. First, couples where 'a one-man woman sleeps only with her one-woman man' never catch any truly sexually transmitted disease (STD, or venereal disease, as it used to be called). Second, the pill does make it easier to have sex in a casual way, perhaps with less commitment. Third, the pill has tended to replace the sheath, and the sheath is quite an effective barrier to the catching or passing on of STDs.

The pill offers some protection against some types of STD, but not enough (page 120); it is thus often blamed for the epidemic the world is now experiencing. To the extent that it has removed one of the important deterrents to copulation without commitment to your partner—fear of an unwanted pregnancy—there must be some truth in this. But how keen we always are to find a scapegoat for the ills of society. The pill does not *cause* STDs: people do, by catching them from each other.

It is a very common myth that people who get these diseases were not careful enough in choosing their partner; and that if you are particularly 'clean' and 'choosy' you will be able to avoid them. Unfortunately, this is not so. STDs cross all geographical and social barriers. They can and do afflict government ministers, doctors, and nurses, just as much as dustmen, cleaners, and dockyard workers and their partners. You may in fact have been very selective as to your partner; but if he or she has had intercourse just once with someone infected with STD, then you too could be infected. Putting it another way, STDs are spread now not so much by the 'professional' as by the enthusiastic amateur.

Why do we no longer refer to 'venereal disease'?

This name is now old fashioned as it only refers officially to two diseases, syphilis and gonorrhoea, with (usually) the addition of one or perhaps two others, depending on the laws of the particular country. Yet the list of infections which can be transmitted in this way is increasing all the time and at the last count there were over 25. They are now nearly as common as colds and influenza. Some of them are almost never caught any other way than by sexual contact. Others, such as a particular form of liver disease (Hepatitis B), are sometimes passed on in other ways though often caught through sex.

What are the symptoms of sexually transmitted diseases?

One of the main problems is that the diseases frequently cause no symptoms at all, especially in women. This means that no one should wait for symptoms before seeking advice if they know, or discover, that they have been exposed to this risk. A *vaginal discharge* in the woman, or a *discharge from the penis* in the man, are the two commonest symptoms. If a woman discovers that her male partner has a discharge, then she has very likely also picked up a form of STD and both partners should go to an STD clinic.

In women, *pain in the lower abdomen*, severe but different from period pains and specially bad with love-making, can be due to pelvic infection (which is often due to STD) whether or not there is also a discharge. *If in doubt, if either has taken a risk, both partners should seek advice*, ideally from an STD clinic which specializes in these diseases (see Useful addresses, page 298). Treatment is entirely confidential, and you do not require a letter of referral from your doctor.

Urethritis can also occur in both sexes. This means inflammation of the tube which conveys urine from the bladder, and is one cause of a *burning pain* on passing water. This does not necessarily mean a sexual infection; it is more likely if the symptom occurs in a man, or in either sex if there is also a discharge.

The fourth most common symptom is a *sore or ulcer*, on the penis in the male, or in the vagina or outside on the vulva in the female. Such sores can be painful if due to the herpes virus, a modern scourge causing recurrent attacks which are infectious each time. A painless sore must on no account be disregarded as it could be due to syphilis. *Warts* on the genitals in either sex can also be acquired sexually. They mean 'get a check-up' just as much as the other symptoms—see below.

Discharges, sores, and warts can sometimes cause irritation or itching but the symptoms may be so minimal that there is a great temptation to do nothing about them. For the sake of your future health and, in women, because pelvic infections due to chlamydia and other STDs can sometimes block up your uterine tubes and so prevent you ever having a baby, it is essential not to attempt any form of self-treatment. Take expert advice if there is the slightest doubt. It may be you have only noticed vaginal warts. But one of the important things about STDs is that they 'hunt in packs': meaning that if you have one which is not serious you could also have picked up something much more important at the same time. Six out of ten women with warts were found to have some other STD as well; and half of all women with gonorrhoea or chlamydia have no symptoms. *It is essential* to have all the tests recommended by the clinic; to continue to the end of any course of treatment, even if you feel well; to report any new symptoms such as *rashes*; and to help the clinic to trace and treat your partner and any other contacts.

Last but not least, remember that there is no immunity after an attack of most STDs. You can be cured of gonorrhoea in the morning with the right antibiotic treatment and catch it again the same evening. But the good news is that with early and correct treatment almost all the *non-viral* sexually transmitted infections are entirely curable.

AIDS—the exception

This disease is caused by the human immunodeficiency virus (HIV) and is 'bad news' in almost every respect. It is fatal, because it destroys the body's ability to fight off infections; it is incurable; and there is no vaccine against it. Everyone who acquires HIV, the virus, has it on board for life, is infectious to others while seeming perfectly healthy for years, but will nearly always get AIDS itself in the end. Almost the only good thing: it is impossible to catch the virus by ordinary social contact, so there is no justification for not being normally friendly in every way with anyone who is infected.

For practical purposes you can assume that the virus can only be transmitted by blood (e.g. sharing needles), by anal or vaginal intercourse, or directly from a mother to her baby in the womb. So once you know the facts HIV is totally avoidable. To quote Dr Malcolm Potts of Family Health International: 'The good news is that no-one need get it—but the bad news is that no-one knows who's got it.'

The only means of self-protection are abstinence, monogamy, and safer sex. *Monogamy* (being loyal to one's loyal partner) has, to quote Claire Rayner's pocket book *Safe Sex*, 'a lot going for it'.

It is far from romantic flimflam to say that the happiest lives are likely to be built on a relationship that has moved from slow and gentle courtship, taking each sexual step one at a time and slowly, rather than in the all-at-once bound that has been fashionable for the last few years, to permanent commitment sealed with a public statement of some kind [like a wedding in fact]. . . . It's a pity that so many of the people who try to encourage monogamy do it in such a finger-wagging hellfire style. . . . We are, by and large, a practical, intelligent lot and we don't like to be bullied. But give us good reasons for a course of action and most of us will accept and change our behaviour accordingly. That is why a lot of people are going to opt for lifelong monogamy as a lifestyle, because they have realised that not only does it protect them from nasty diseases that can and do shorten life; it can also be fun and comfortable and make you feel secure.

And, I would add, if things become as bad in the world of straight heterosexual sex as the World Health Organization predicts, *monogamous sex will in future be the only truly 'fun sex' in which 'anything goes' between two people who love each other*. Outside, sex will be a bit scary, less fun, requiring the use of condoms and virucides with no certainty that the infection won't still get across.

However in the real world many if not most people are faithful within each relationship, but they do change partners at more or less frequent intervals. This is often called 'serial monogamy'. The problem is that any new partner brings with him or her all the chances of infection represented directly or indirectly by all those they have ever slept with: if someone has just eight partners who have had eight partners who have had eight partners . . . even stopping there (and in practice the contacts go much further) means over 500 chances of being linked with the killer virus. For this life-style, *safer sex* means (a) discovering all the ways of pleasuring each other which avoid contact with the relevant body fluids (semen, vaginal fluids, and blood) and (b) otherwise *using condoms; even if using (say) the pill for contraception.*

Finally, two more quotes from Malcolm Potts:

Those at greatest risk are those in their late teens and early 20s who are the most sexually active and who often believe themselves immortal. If education is to work it must convince them (1) that they are at risk (2) that a lethal disease can be completely without symptoms and (3) that safer sex offers worthwhile protection.

And on risk-taking:

Risk-taking and AIDS are not unlike risk-taking and pregnancy. Neither AIDS infection nor fertilization are certain, the gambler often survives, and the penalty is remote: nine months in the case of pregnancy, maybe years in the case of AIDS.

See Further reading for more about STDs (page 291).

Cancer of the cervix (entrance to the uterus)
It is very interesting that modern research shows that this cancer, along with the earliest cell changes before it develops, behaves rather like an STD. It is probably spread sexually by a virus or combination of viruses. The main microscopic type of this cancer never occurs in a woman who has not had intercourse. It is far more common in women who have sex first when they are very young (under the age of 16) and who have had many different partners. *If this applies to you do not panic.* Nature gives an early warning of future trouble, which can be found in cervical smears (page 81). Actual cancer is then preventable by minor treatment, usually as an out-patient. Even if in your area the policy is for routine smears every five or every three years, you should ask the doctor in confidence whether to have them more often because of your sexual history. Most experts recommend annual smears if you have had herpes or wart virus infections (also risk factors), and certainly if previous smears have ever been abnormal.

More about the pill and responsibility in sex

Some people think that the only things that show whether somebody has been sexually responsible are if he or she has (a) not caused an unwanted pregnancy and (b) not acquired a sexually transmitted disease. Both are worthwhile aims—a little negative perhaps, but good. Yet *the good can sometimes be an enemy of the best*. Making love is something special, definitely not for throwing around. It is nature's physical 'seal of approval' on a loving and caring relationship between two people. Deep down, everyone knows that a sexual experience which pre-dates a loving experience is a pale shadow of the real thing. Consider this quote from Dr Esther Sapire (see Further reading):

Sex is part of oneself to accept and live with comfortably and enjoy. It is not something that comes in from outside and takes over the body and flies off. It is something we *are* not something we *do* as a physical act and it cannot be isolated from the total relationship. Sex is an expression of love, and is only one aspect of it which enhances the relationship. . . . There is a time when one is ready for sexual experiences, but if the process is hastened unduly without allowing the natural process to 'unfold' at its own pace, it may never function well. This can be likened to a closed, exquisite rosebud being pulled open by someone impatient to see it in its full glory—only to find the petals bruised and torn in the process, and that it does not fulfil its potential of giving pleasure.

Many can confirm that love-making is actually more fun and more exciting if the couple care for and trust each other: if in fact they are 'in love'. Love says 'What can I give?' much more than 'What can I get?' *As a minimum*, I think that responsible sex means asking these three questions before any couple make love: 'Do we want, and can we care for, a baby?'; 'If not, are we using a reliable method of family planning, such as the pill?'; and most important, 'Will making love with this person lead to anyone, my partner, myself, or any third party, being hurt?' Having realized that someone might very well get hurt, some people actually decide not to have sex (before they are sure they have met 'Mr or Miss Right', for example, or outside of a long-term relationship) *even with precautions*. They are using what has been described as the 'safest of all oral contraceptives', namely the word 'No' . . . They do after all have rights over their own body and, to quote Esther Sapire again, 'they can *choose* when and by whom to be touched without shame or guilt, and they have the right to say "No" if they so desire without feeling old fashioned or freakish.' Worth a thought.

Oddly enough, sociological research has regularly shown that so-called *integrated* relationships with sharing and communication have a much better track record for avoiding an unwanted pregnancy than do the non-sharing often short-term *segregated* type. Couples in integrated relationships consider and discuss contraception as part and parcel of their sexual relationship. So it is arranged first. Contraception in segregated relationships is seen as entirely the woman's business, and she gets around to it *after* sex starts happening, if then. Connected with this is another well-established fact, that *most unplanned*

conceptions happen at the start and at the end of relationships.
At the start, couples without good lines of communication are
often inhibited from actually discussing contraception. And at a
'bust-up' there seems no point in continuing to take the pill; but
often there is at least one attempt at reconciliation along with
sex—and the sheath is either not available or seems truly a
'barrier'. Whatever the explanation, those are the times when
most unwanted conceptions happen. If so there's a pretty
obvious conclusion, but vanishingly few experts in this area are
prepared to come out with it. If unwanted conception is a
feature of the start and finish of relationships, much better
on contraceptive grounds to have loyal, long-term, relationships
and thus fewer contraceptively dangerous partner changes!

Should we not think about whether . . . it is family planning clinics we
really need? Perhaps 'relationship clinics', welcoming young men and
young women, would be more appropriate, with the dispensing of
contraception an important, though subsidiary, function. (Carolynne
Skinner, *The British Journal of Family Planning*, 1985 (11), 60–2.)

What about the pill in all this? It cannot be expected to be a
cure-all of society's ills. Nor should it be blamed for too many
of them—they are caused by people, not by the pill. Certainly it
can enable some people to behave irresponsibly, people who
forget that bodies also have feelings and emotions attached.
Even then, at least a disastrous pregnancy will be avoided. A
child has the best chance in life if born to parents who trust
each other and are prepared to keep *working* on their
relationship, so as to ensure an emotionally secure and happy
home for all the years he or she needs to reach maturity.

I believe that pill prescribers, whatever their own religious
and moral views, should meet and counsel the person or couple
requesting contraception on their own ground. Consider the
following analogy. If I were a Jehovah's Witness, it would be
immoral for me to receive a blood transfusion. Yet, as a
doctor, I could feel that it was right for me to transfuse a
dangerously ill patient who did not share my views, *on his or
her say-so*.

Thus prescribers of the pill need not betray their own
principles while refraining from forcing them on others. They

should have come to terms with their own sexuality and should be as good at listening as at talking, though prepared to say a 'word in season' based on the first paragraph of this section if (and only if) appropriate. They should be equipped to give helpful counselling, particularly for those who are immature, emotionally, whatever their age in years. Prescribers should be specially sensitive too to those with inhibitions of whatever kind, for example some who may have guilt feelings about sex, or about family planning. Everyone is different.

2

....

The pill: how does it work?

The idea of an oral contraceptive has been around for at least two thousand years. But nothing very useful came out of centuries of magic and mumbo-jumbo plus a great deal of trial and error. It was only when the normal processes of male and female reproduction were better understood that scientists could begin to devise more effective methods for blocking them.

The normal menstrual cycle

During their fertile years women are unique in having a more or less regular cycle of changes in their bodies. This cycle is caused by the ebb and flow in the bloodstream of various hormones or chemical messengers which are released into it by certain glands. The whole process is controlled by the brain, as is shown by the well-known fact that if a woman has a stressful emotional upset her periods can stop altogether for months at a time. Parts of the brain which are particularly involved have special names (such as the preoptic area and the hypothalamus), but I shall here call them simply the 'base of the brain'.

As you can see in Figure 5, just below the base of the brain is the pituitary gland, sometimes called the 'leader of the hormone orchestra' because it is so important. Yet it is really quite small, just the size of a large pea. The ovaries and uterus are the other main parts of the system and are also shown. Blood flows through them all connecting the whole system together. Any hormone released into the blood by one gland can therefore travel to all the others and can cause its own specific effects there or as appropriate anywhere in the whole body.

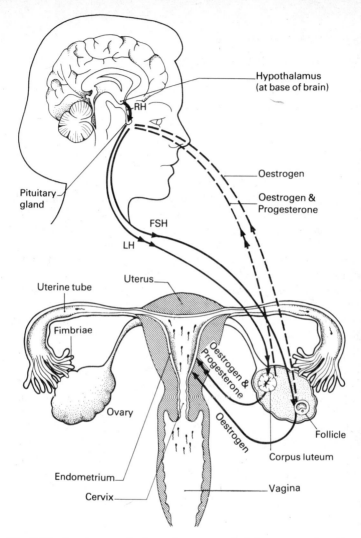

Fig. 5 The female reproductive system: control of the menstrual cycle

Notes: 1. Single arrowhead ▶ relates to events of the first half of the cycle (follicular phase). Double arrowheads ▶ ▶ relate to the second half (luteal phase).

2. Dotted lines show feedback effects (see pages 39–40).

3. RH = releasing hormone; FSH = follicle stimulating hormone; LH = luteinizing hormone.

Egg-release from the ovaries

The ovaries are about the same size as a peach-stone, though much less hard. Like the testicle of a man they have two functions: the production and release of special sex cells (in this case eggs) and of hormones into the bloodstream. There are literally millions of potential egg cells in the ovaries of a baby girl before birth, but by the age of puberty the number has dropped to only 200,000. Yet there will be no shortage. Normally only one egg is released from one or other ovary during each menstrual cycle which commonly lasts for 28 days. Thus only about 13 are required each year. As no woman can be fertile for more than a maximum of about 40 years, only something over 500 eggs will ever be required. Occasionally, of course, more than one egg is released, leading if pregnancy follows to twins or perhaps triplets. The egg is released from the largest out of several fluid-filled balloons or egg-sacs called follicles and is picked up by the seaweed-like fronds (or fimbriae) of the outer end of one of the uterine (Fallopian) tubes: see Figure 6. It then starts its journey down the uterine tube, partly by the whole tube contracting and partly because there are microscopic paddles (cilia) within it which beat rhythmically in the direction of the uterus.

This happens about the middle of a cycle, if it is going to be four weeks in length. The time from egg-release (often called ovulation) to the start of the next period is the only part of the cycle which is fixed in length and lasts 14 days. Many quite normal cycles last less or more than the usual 28 days. If so the variability is almost all in the length of the first phase of the cycle from the start of the period up to egg-release. The first day of menstrual bleeding is always called day 1 of the cycle. So if, for example, a woman has a 35-day cycle, egg-release happens on day (35 − 14 =) 21.

The cycle occurs because of a marvellously controlled interaction of hormones. The most important ones are two produced by the pituitary gland—follicle stimulating hormone (FSH) and luteinizing hormone (LH)—and two from the ovaries—oestrogen and progesterone. Up to the time of egg-release, the ovary produces only the one female hormone called

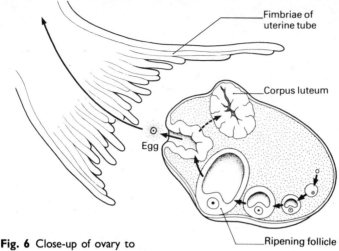

Fimbriae of
uterine tube

Corpus luteum

Egg

Ripening follicle

Fig. 6 Close-up of ovary to
show growth of follicles and
formation of corpus luteum
after egg-release.

oestrogen. It is made in cells within the walls of the follicles,
depicted in Figure 6. These give their name to the first part of
the menstrual cycle, the follicular phase. During the second part
of the menstrual cycle, for almost exactly 14 days, the particular
empty follicle from which the egg came that month now
produces another hormone called progesterone as well as
oestrogen. It also turns yellow in colour, and so is given the
name corpus luteum (which just means 'yellow body' in Latin),
and this part of the cycle is called the luteal phase (see Figure
7a). The name luteinizing hormone for the hormone which
causes this change means no more than 'the yellow-making
hormone'.

The uterus

These hormones travel to the uterus during both phases of the
cycle. Their main business there is to thicken its lining with
extra glandular tissue and blood-vessels so that it is ready just in

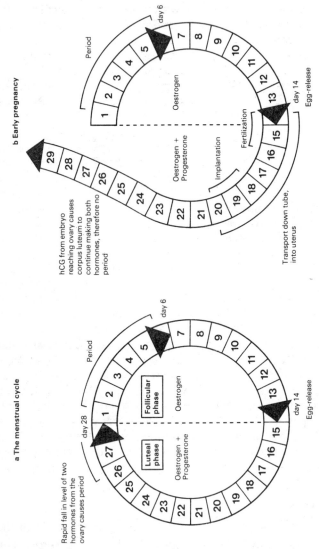

a The menstrual cycle

Period

day 28

day 6

Rapid fall in level of two hormones from the ovary causes period

Follicular phase

Luteal phase

Oestrogen

Oestrogen + Progesterone

day 14

Egg-release

b Early pregnancy

Period

day 6

Oestrogen

Oestrogen + Progesterone

day 14

Egg-release

Fertilization

Implantation

Transport down tube, into uterus

hCG from embryo reaching ovary causes corpus luteum to continue making both hormones, therefore no period

Fig. 7 (a) The menstrual cycle (b) Early pregnancy

Note: Assumes standard 28-day cycle. Follicular phase is the part that varies, if the actual cycle is longer or shorter than 28 days.

case a pregnancy starts that month. If the woman has recently had unprotected sex, a sperm may reach the egg in the uterine tube and join up with it. This is fertilization. The fertilized egg starts just 14-hundredths of a millimetre in size. It begins to divide on its journey along the uterine tube towards the uterus, and embeds itself in the prepared lining around the nineteenth day of the cycle. This is called implantation (Figure 7b).

The embryo, as the early pregnancy is called, now has just over a week to prevent the next period happening. This is vital, otherwise it will be washed out by the menstrual flow. It does this by itself producing a special hormone, whose name is human chorionic gonadotrophin (hCG). This sends an urgent message in the bloodstream to the yellow body, the corpus luteum, to make sure it keeps on producing its hormones (oestrogen and progesterone). These therefore keep coming in the blood to the uterus, and ensure that the lining of the uterus is not shed, so it can continue to provide nourishment for the developing embryo (Figure 7b). Considering this intricate series of events, it is remarkable that a fully formed human being ever results.

Menstruation: the period

In fact, implantation very often fails—probably in over one-third of cases (see page 236). Or the egg was never fertilized. Either way, the preparations for pregnancy come to nothing. The ovary stops producing oestrogen and progesterone as regularly at about 14 days after egg-release as if it had a timing mechanism programmed to switch it off. This rapid loss of the hormones which produce and maintain the lining of the uterus causes it to break down and leave the body through the cervix and vagina (Figure 5). This causes the bleeding of the first day of the next period, which is day 1 of the *next* menstrual cycle (see Figure 7a).

The pituitary gland

Just as hormones from the ovary control what happens in the uterus, so the hormones from the pituitary gland tell the ovary to produce the correct hormones for each phase of the cycle. One of them, luteinizing hormone (LH), is released in large amounts at mid-cycle, and this signal is what actually triggers off the bursting of the largest follicle to release an egg. This signal is never given in pregnancy because enough of the hormones oestrogen and progesterone comes from the ovary to the pituitary gland to 'switch it off'. This prevents any further eggs being released and so explains why a woman who is already pregnant cannot go on getting pregnancies in the next nine months.

The pill

The combined oral contraceptive pill contains similar hormones to the oestrogen and progesterone produced by the ovary. Hence the pituitary gland is, as you might say, 'fooled' into thinking the woman is already pregnant. From its point of view, there is no need to send out hormones to stimulate the ovaries if there are already high levels of ovarian-type hormones. So the pituitary cuts drastically its output of the hormones FSH and LH. In particular there are no more of those mid-cycle 'surges' of a large amount of LH which are essential for egg-release. With so little of the hormones from the pituitary reaching them, the ovaries also go into a resting state, and produce minimal amounts of natural oestrogen and progesterone. Both the pituitary and the ovaries are like factories where the main production line has stopped, perhaps for a works' holiday, but small-scale production and essential maintenance are continuing. Such a factory can start full-scale production at short notice as soon as the work-force returns. Similarly, when a woman discontinues the pill, the hormone factories in the pituitary and ovaries rapidly return to normal working.

While a woman is taking the pill the normal menstrual cycle stops altogether. However, 'periods' of a sort are still produced, because the artificial hormones in the pill do have some effect on the lining of the uterus. When they are removed for one week out of every four this rather thinner lining comes away along with some bleeding. See page 47 for more details about this.

So much for a brief summary of the menstrual cycle and how the pill works. Continue reading here if you would like a more detailed account, but otherwise you may like to skip to page 42.

*More about the menstrual cycle

*The follicular phase

In order to start each new cycle, a special hormone called the releasing hormone (RH) travels from the base of the brain and causes the pituitary gland to release follicle stimulating hormone (FSH). See Figure 5; you will find it helpful to keep referring to this and to Figure 7 throughout this section. FSH travels in the blood to the ovaries. Its main action, as its name implies, is to stimulate the growth of some of the many thousands of follicles which are contained in each ovary. Follicles are tiny, thick-walled, fluid-filled egg-sacs, each lined by a layer of cells which are capable of producing hormones, and also containing an immature egg cell (oocyte). FSH usually stimulates about twenty of these follicles to grow, and also causes the lining cells to start to manufacture oestrogen and release it into the blood. One particular follicle in one or other ovary is stimulated to grow and to 'ripen' more than all the others. Its egg cell is also maturing, ready to be released and, should it get the chance, to be fertilized.

Oestrogens arc the fundamentally female hormones which influence the whole body, producing rounded contours, breast development, and many other features of femininity. They also stimulate the uterus to grow its new lining to replace the one that was shed at the previous menstrual period. The lining is made of many little glands, set in several layers of cells which also contain arteries and veins. Oestrogen makes the glands grow and the layers of intervening cells increase.

Meanwhile the rising levels of oestrogen in the blood have been having a most important effect back on the base of the brain and the pituitary gland. This is known as 'negative feedback' and it is important to understand this if you are to understand clearly how the pill works.

In general terms, negative feedback means that if the level of a hormone in the blood goes *up*, the level of the stimulating hormone which *caused* it to go up is made to go *down*.

In the menstrual cycle, this means for example:

up ↑ oestrogen in blood causes *down* ↓ FSH

The opposite is also true:

down ↓ oestrogen in blood causes *up* ↑ FSH

Engineers call this a servo-mechanism.

So at the stage of the menstrual cycle we have now reached the rise in the level of oestrogen causes over several days a fall in the pituitary gland's output of its FSH.

By about the thirteenth day of a standard 28-day cycle the stimulated follicles have produced a rise of oestrogen in the blood to a peak level up to six times higher than it was on the first day. By negative feedback this has caused the level of the stimulating hormone FSH to drop. Now a most interesting and crucially different thing happens. Once the amount of oestrogen reaching the pituitary gland gets to a critical level, it releases into the bloodstream a sudden surge of luteinizing hormone (LH). In other words, the *rise* in oestrogen is now causing a *rise* of a hormone from the pituitary. This is called 'positive feedback', to distinguish it from the negative type which operates all the rest of the time throughout the menstrual cycle.

This large amount of LH is conveyed by the blood to the active ovary. This is the one containing the largest follicle, now a balloon bulging the surface of the ovary and about 2 centimetres in diameter. The main job of this surge of LH is to cause the balloon to burst, resulting in ovulation and the release of a now mature and fertilizable egg. If all goes well, this is picked up by the fimbriae of the uterine tube and transported towards the uterus (see Figure 6). As this occurs some women notice in their lower abdomen, on one or other side, a variable amount of pain which is given the German name Mittelschmerz.

Once the egg has been released, the follicle collapses and becomes that bright yellow body, the corpus luteum. Along with the change in colour of the cells lining its wall there is a change in what they do. As well as continuing to produce oestrogen, for the first time these luteal cells start to manufacture and release into the blood a new hormone called progesterone.

The luteal phase

Progesterone, like oestrogen, has effects all over the body and, for instance, is responsible for the slight rise in body temperature during the second half of the cycle which is the basis for the temperature method of family planning. But its main effect is on the lining of the uterus, to prepare it for a pregnancy. Indeed the word progesterone means 'pro-gestation: in favour of child-bearing'. It thickens the lining of the uterus still further and causes its glands to release a nutritious fluid. Now if a sperm successfully fertilizes an egg, the resulting pre-embryo travels down the tube and about five days after egg-release begins to embed itself in that lining. This embedding process is called implantation. It is not complete until the fourteenth day (the day the next period would be due). The embryo produces hCG, a hormone which so exactly copies the action of LH from the pituitary (page 37) that it prolongs the life of the corpus luteum in the ovary. This ensures that it continues to produce sufficent progesterone and oestrogen. After about five weeks from ovulation the placenta (afterbirth) produces enough of these two vital hormones to maintain the pregnancy. As long as they continue to be produced, from either source, there will be no menstrual flow and the embryo can remain secure within the lining of the uterus. A second effect of these two hormones, working in concert, is to lower the amounts of LH and FSH released from the pituitary by the more usual negative feedback process. This is important, as it prevents any more surges of LH.

If, however, a sperm fails to reach the egg on its way down the tube, the egg ceases to be fertilizable very quickly, about 12 hours after ovulation. For reasons which are still not clear, the corpus luteum abruptly ceases to function twelve to fourteen days after it was first formed, unless hCG from a developing embryo dictates differently. There is therefore a rapid fall in the levels of both oestrogen and progesterone. This has two results: first, by negative feedback, the amount of RH coming from the base of the brain to the pituitary increases and therefore the amount of FSH released increases. When this extra FSH in the blood reaches the ovaries, another group of 20 or so follicles are stimulated to grow, one of them being destined to release its

The pill: how does it work?   41

egg during the *next* normal menstrual cycle. Second, the sudden fall in the levels of both oestrogen and progesterone in the bloodstream reaching the uterus causes local changes in its now thick lining which lead to it being shed during a normal menstrual period. How heavy and how long the bleeding during the first few days of the next cycle is varies considerably. Substances called prostaglandins are involved in this process: one of their effects is to ensure that the uterus contracts to expel the blood, but this can also cause menstrual cramping pain (dysmenorrhoea) which can be severe in some women.

The description I have just given is still simplified. 'Oestrogen' is in fact a family of hormones, the most important member of which in the menstrual cycle is oestradiol. The 'surge' of LH is accompanied by a smaller surge of FSH. Releasing hormone (RH) normally reaches the pituitary in an intermittent, so-called pulsatile fashion, and this important mechanism is disturbed by progesterone (or any progestogen). Another hormone from the pituitary gland called prolactin is involved; and the whole cycle can be affected by quite different hormones such as those from the thyroid gland, as well as by the nervous system.

How the pill was developed

To recap: so long as there are reasonably high levels of the two hormones oestrogen and progesterone, the base of the brain and the pituitary gland are kept inactive (by negative feedback). This prevents:

(a) release of sufficient FSH to ripen any follicles in preparation for egg-release;

(b) any surges of LH, without which the actual process of release of an egg is impossible.

These results are regularly produced by the high levels of both the natural hormones during the second half of the normal menstrual cycle and throughout any pregnancy.

That the corpus luteum of pregnancy stops further egg-release was first shown in the early 1900s. In 1921 the Austrian Dr Haberlandt was the first scientist on record to suggest that extracts from the ovaries of pregnant animals might be used as oral contraceptives. It was in fact from extracts of either the corpus luteum or the follicles of rat ovaries that progesterone and several different oestrogens were isolated and eventually each chemical formula was determined.

By the late 1930s Dr Rock and Dr Kurzrok in America, among others, were beginning to use the hormones in both fertile and infertile women. As Dr Haberlandt had predicted, and some researchers using rabbits had shown, these hormones could be used to stop egg-release.

However, natural progesterone and oestrogens were not satisfactory when given by mouth since they are largely destroyed in the digestive system. In these experiments they had to be given by injection. In 1939 Inhoffen in Germany managed to produce an oestrogen which could be taken orally. It was called ethinyloestradiol, but over 20 years were to pass before it became one of the two oestrogens used in combined pills. The other is called mestranol.

The other main problem in the 1930s and early 1940s was that the raw material for all steroid hormones had to be extracted from animal sources. To produce just 12 mg of oestradiol, for example, required the ovaries of 80,000 sows. This made the hormones fearfully expensive. The next breakthrough came in 1943 when an eccentric American chemist called Russell Marker managed to produce pure progesterone from diosgenin extracted from wild Mexican yams.

Using the same raw material, a team led by George Rosenkranz and Carl Djerassi then produced the first orally active progestogen, norethisterone, in 1951. In North America this is known as norethindrone, and until very recently it was the most widely used progestogen in the world. Working independently, two years later Dr Frank Colton in Chicago produced a very similar progestogen called norethynodrel—the main one used in the early contraceptive drug trials.

The stage was now set for the development of the pill as we know it. But many pharmaceutical companies feared the controversy that might result and were reluctant to apply these hormones for contraception, though they were happy for them to be used in the treatment of various gynaecological conditions. Margaret Sanger, with her wealthy friend Catherine McCormack, provided the encouragement and resources to researchers that eventually led to the marketing of the pill. The leaders of this work were the biologists Gregory Pincus and H. C. Chang, and the obstetrician John Rock. They worked first with animals and then used a small group of human volunteers in Boston. It soon became clear that the new hormones were very effective contraceptives, and produced no immediate or obvious harmful effects.

Trials with a larger number of women began in Puerto Rico in 1956, supervised by a young gynaecologist called Celso Ramón-Garcia and Edris Rice-Wray (the first female physician involved in testing the pill). The trials were highly successful—until that is, the chemists got rid of an impurity in the pills. This impurity was the oestrogen, mestranol. Immediately things began to go wrong. Irregular bleeding occurred and so did accidental pregnancies. So it was really by chance that the researchers learnt that a little oestrogen was necessary for maximum effectiveness and control of the cycle. When they put it back in the amount previously present as an 'impurity', the combined pill was created. It took a few more years until June 1960 for the US Food and Drug Administration to release the first combination oestrogen and progestogen birth control pill Enavid-10. This contained what we would now consider far higher doses of the hormones than necessary or advisable. It is a fact that early pills gave as much oestrogen in a day as is now taken in a week, and as much progestogen (norethisterone) as one current pill provides in a whole month!

It was agreed from the start that these new and powerful medicines should be distributed only under close supervision and the initial recommendation was that they should not be used for more than two years continuously. That idea, of using the pill only for a very few years at a time, has persisted in many people's thinking—dubiously in the light of all the facts (page 151). The pill seemed to be safe but there was no certainty that it would prove to be so in the long term. Yet it was so much more acceptable than all previous methods of reversible family planning that women all over the world took to using it sooner and in greater numbers than almost anyone expected.

Since then newer and better progestogens have been devised

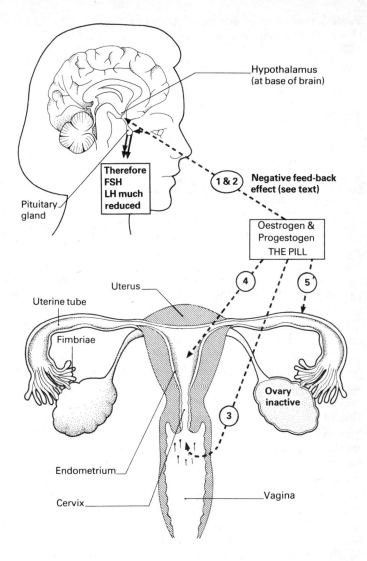

Fig. 8 How the combined pill prevents pregnancy

Note: Numbers 1–5 are the contraceptive effects of the combined pill as shown in Table 2.

Table 2 How combined pills prevent pregnancy
(The more +s means the greater the effect)

	'Ordinary' combined pills
1. Reduced FSH therefore follicles stopped from ripening and egg from maturing	++++
2. LH surge stopped so no egg-release	++++
3. Cervical mucus changed into a barrier to sperm	+++
4. Lining of uterus made less suitable for implantation of an embryo	+++
5. Uterine tubes perhaps affected so that they do not transport egg so well (uncertainty about this)	+
Expected pregnancy rate per 100 women using the pill method for one year (compare use of NO METHOD = 80–90)	0.2 to 1

Note: The combined pill is *very* reliable with plenty of back-up effects—but relies chiefly on effects 1 and 2. See Table 11 (page 208) for the progestogen-only pill.

(page 155), and Mexican yams are no longer required for the raw material. But ethinyloestradiol as the oestrogen has not yet been bettered.

Figure 8 and Table 2 show the ways by which the usual combined pill operates to prevent pregnancy. The main effect is to stop the normal hormone changes of the menstrual cycle and hence prevent both maturing of follicles and ovulation—points 1 and 2 in the Table. However, there are several back-up mechanisms to make pregnancy unlikely even if egg-release should occur. (The commonest reason for this 'breakthrough' egg-release is forgetting to take tablets.) These back-up mechanisms are shown in the Figure and Table. The slippery mucus which normally flows from the cervix in the middle of the cycle and at that time is easily penetrated by sperm is transformed by the hormones—actually the progestogen—into a scanty, thick material which produces a quite effective barrier to sperm. There are also changes in the lining of the uterus which seem to make it less able to support and nourish a fertilized egg. Finally, though this is more debatable, the tubes may perhaps function less well in conveying the egg towards the uterus, perhaps making it less likely to survive even if it were fertilized.

Effectiveness against pregnancy

There is no more effective reversible method of family planning than the combined pill. This is probably because its back-up systems as just described can operate even if the prime effect of preventing release of an egg from the ovary were to fail. But failures do occur for two reasons: failures of the method (which are rare) and failures of the user (forgetting tablets: not so rare). If these two causes of failure are added together, the total failure rate can be around 1 per 100 woman-years. What does this mean? The simple explanation is that if 100 women used the pill for a year, one of them should expect to get pregnant. Put another way, if you the user were to be fertile for 100 years, you would have an 'evens' chance of one pregnancy at the end of that time! Impossible, of course, but it gives the general idea. For healthy women who take their pills absolutely regularly at the same time every day, the failure rate is reduced about fivefold, to as low as 0.2 per 100 woman-years with modern pills. This means just two pregnancies among 1,000 users per year. You would have to be fertile for 500 years (!) before you would have an evens chance of one pregnancy . . . However, that one failure *could* of course happen in the very first year rather than the five hundredth.

In practice, methods which depend on great care by the users, like the sheath and the diaphragm, have overall (user) failure rates of about 10 per 100 woman-years. On average this means one unplanned pregnancy every 10 years. Couples should perhaps work out the implications of this statistic more when planning their final family size . . .

What causes 'periods' on the combined pill?

When the pill is taken the normal menstrual cycle is abolished. Just so long as sufficient of the artificial oestrogen and progestogen of the pill are in the bloodstream there will be no bleeding from the uterus. However, most women like to see some kind of period, as regular reassurance that the pill is working. It may also be better to reduce the monthly intake of

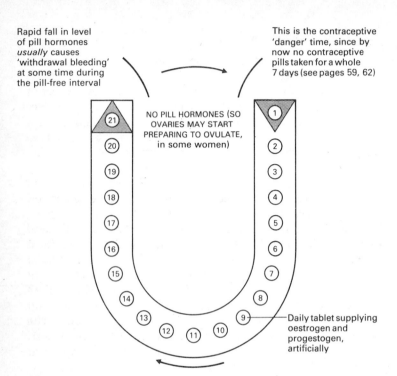

Rapid fall in level of pill hormones *usually* causes 'withdrawal bleeding' at some time during the pill-free interval

This is the contraceptive 'danger' time, since by now no contraceptive pills taken for a whole 7 days (see pages 59, 62)

NO PILL HORMONES (SO OVARIES MAY START PREPARING TO OVULATE, in some women)

Daily tablet supplying oestrogen and progestogen, artificially

Fig. 9 The pill cycle (21-day system)

Note: Compare with Figure 7a (page 36). The normal cycle shown there is taken right away and *replaced* by this simpler one. The bleeding from the uterus is caused just by withdrawal of the pill hormones.

Pill-taking is drawn in a horseshoe for the important reason that *a horseshoe is a symmetrical object*. Hence the pill-free interval can be lengthened, leading to the risk of conception, either side of the horseshoe: by forgetting pills either at the beginning *or* at the end of the packet. See text, pages 58–66.

artificial hormones to a minimum, and to give the pituitary and ovaries and one's body chemistry generally (page 86) a break from time to time from the actions of the pill hormones. Solely for these reasons, most systems of pill-taking include a pill-free time, usually a week in every 28 days. The effect of thus cutting off the supply of pill hormones is to *imitate* the fall in the levels in the bloodstream of their natural equivalents at the end of a normal cycle. This causes shedding of the rather thinner lining of the uterus which the pill's hormones have produced during the previous 21 days (see Figure 9). Because the lining is different—caused in a different way, by the pill, and looking different under the microscope—its shedding usually leads to less bleeding, often darker in colour, than a normal menstrual period. It is also a lot less likely to be painful.

So if you are on the pill your normal cycle is removed and replaced by something different. You are causing the 'periods' yourself by stopping the pills for one week out of every four. You could stop having periods altogether any time, if you in fact made no break from pill-taking. *As they are in reality substitute periods*, they are often more accurately called *hormone withdrawal bleeds*.

An important conclusion from all this is that if for some reason they fail to happen on the pill, it probably only means that there was too little artificially produced lining of the uterus that month for the stopping of the pill's hormones to lead to bleeding. 'Bad blood' is not 'piling up inside'. There just is *no blood to come away*. If you have been taking your pills regularly the explanation is very unlikely to be pregnancy. (If in doubt this can be confirmed by a test.) What is more, *absence of hormone withdrawal bleeds is totally irrelevant to any risk to your future chances of having a baby* (page 127).

How unnatural is the pill?

People are often concerned that even if it did not have unwanted side-effects (which I am going to discuss in some detail) the pill's main contraceptive effect in suppressing the cyclical activities of the ovary and of the pituitary gland is 'unnatural'. But is it? Surely having menstrual cycles and periods is actually not entirely 'natural'. Biologically, suppression of the menstrual cycle for years at a time may in fact be a much more natural state of affairs. In the past, before there was effective contraception, the normal thing was for a woman to be either pregnant or breast-feeding during all the child-bearing years. A doctor working in Central Africa once told me that he had been visited some years ago by a woman in her early forties who was worried by bleeding. By excluding all the other possibilities, he eventually diagnosed this as a normal period. She had been anxious because she never remembered having such a thing before!

Far from the myth that periods are normal and necessary to 'flush out the flues', they really are not what nature intends.

As support for this notion, it does seem that some cancers, notably cancer of the ovary and the endometrium (lining of the womb), are commoner in women who have had more rather than less natural menstrual cycles during their lives. Probably for this reason, the pill seems to be *protective against these very cancers* (pages 143–4). Can we also be reassured by the fact that the pill's main action is to imitate the corpus luteum of pregnancy? Or that many of the changes in body chemistry caused by the pill (page 86), and not a few of the minor side-effects such as nausea, are so similar to those of pregnancy?

These questions cannot yet be given definite answers. Although in many ways the effects of the pill are similar to those of pregnancy, they are by no means all the same: and pregnancy is anyway not free of risks. What is more, the hormones used are artificial rather than natural. (So far, experiments using natural hormones in the pill have not been very satisfactory, but they are continuing.) The dosage of the two hormones is not exactly tailored to each individual. It is roughly constant for three weeks out of four rather than continuously varying as in the menstrual cycle. (So-called phasic pills (page 192) imitate the menstrual cycle a little more closely, but still not perfectly.) And finally, the fact that some natural hormones are still produced by the woman's ovaries in addition to the artificial ones she is taking by mouth could have some effect.

So the most that should be said is that there are reasons to believe that the pill is *not quite so unnatural* as appears at first sight. In passing, it is a strange fact that some of the people who say the pill is 'unnatural' do something else which is equally unnatural, and on present evidence considerably more dangerous —they smoke cigarettes! The pill contains two substances which are at least similar to hormones the body is used to handling. And pills are eaten—nothing in the animal kingdom takes food or alien chemicals on board through its lungs. The cigarette however is a chemical factory, manufacturing over 2,000 unnatural compounds *which are absorbed via the lungs to travel in the blood all over the body.* Some are known cancer-causing agents.

Research continues, and we certainly know a lot more now about the use of hormones for oral contraception than we did at the time of those early tests in Puerto Rico. Indeed, more is known about the safety of the pill than the majority of drugs or food additives on the market (see page 167). A great deal more money has been spent in safety-testing it than was ever spent in inventing it.

3

....

The pill: how do I take it?

The progestogen-only pill (mini-pill) is considered in Chapter 8.

Systems of pill-taking

The most common system is the one in which you take one pill daily for 21 days followed by a 7-day break. In most countries *'everyday' (ED) brands* are available with 28 tablets in each packet, of which seven are dummies, or 'blanks'. These are liked by many women. Care must be taken when starting these packets to avoid taking dummy pills at the wrong time, but the pills are then taken consecutively, one packet after another. There is no need to remember when to stop and start taking successive courses. They have certain other advantages too (page 62).

There is another way to take pills, called the *three-monthly or 'tricycle' system*. In this, either four or (more usually now) three packets are taken in succession—therefore a pill every day for 63 days—followed by a break during which the 'period' normally occurs. As explained in the last chapter, pill 'periods' are in fact 'hormone withdrawal bleeds', created artificially by the taking of a 7-day break. So there is no particular reason why they should not happen every 10 weeks, with the three packs in a row system, instead of every four weeks. Once this has been explained, many find this four- or five-periods-per-year routine quite acceptable, indeed preferable.

Moreover, there are some special reasons why the doctor may recommend this even without your particular preference:

(a) If *headaches* are a problem and happen in the pill-free week. Tricycling really does help, meaning at most five bad headaches a year instead of 13. This can be the policy even for migraines, so long as they are not the type described on page 101.

(b) If the '*periods*' themselves are bad (unusual on the pill).

(c) In managing epilepsy (page 112).

(d) In treating endometriosis (page 122).

(e) Previous failure of the pill leading to pregnancy. This important reason is discussed in detail on page 183.

A word of caution though: this tricycle system does mean you will need 15–16 packets of pills per year instead of the usual 13. Thus you take more hormones on board and this might tend to increase the risk of some side-effects (page 153). The breaks themselves may also be beneficial, in giving the body a regular 'rest' from the pill's effects (page 151). I therefore recommend that this tricycle scheme is reserved for when there is one of the above special reasons, or of course at the woman's choice after discussion of these pros and cons.

The tricycle system of pill-taking is of course completely different from triphasic pills, which are described on page 192. Indeed, it does not work satisfactorily with any phasic pills: the more common single phase (monophasic) brands need to be used.

Postponing 'periods'

Even if you regularly use the three weeks on, one week off system, one advantage of the pill is that there is no objection on special occasions to your postponing your 'periods'. When planning for your holidays for example, this can be done either by taking extra pills from a spare packet, or more simply by just taking two packets in succession. If you happen to have pill periods always at weekends, a few extra days' pill-taking in one cycle can shift them to mid-week regularly in future. Note, however, that there are special rules for phasic pills (pages 192–6) and that it is *not* recommended that you bring your 'period' on sooner by stopping pill-taking early.

Whenever you take the *7-day break* from pill-taking, your protection against pregnancy continues throughout it, provided three things are true:

(a) you have been regular in your pill-taking from the preceding packet;

(b) none of the other conditions which might reduce your protection has applied in your case (see pages 58–72);

(c) *you do in fact start another packet on the eighth day*.

If (c) is not true, sperm can survive so long, that after love-making on say the sixth or seventh day after the last pill, they could be in the uterine tubes and still fertilize an egg released later, during the following week.

How to start taking the pill

If you are having normal periods up to the time of starting the pill, there are two ways to start. The *now out-of-date method* is to take the first pill on the fifth day of your period, whether your bleeding has stopped or not. Choose a pill from the section on the packet marked with that day of the week and press down on the plastic bubble so as to remove it from the foil on the reverse side. Then take a pill a day for 21 days. After a 7-day break you then start taking pills again on the eighth day: and from then on in each four weeks you follow the regular routine of 21 days of pill-taking followed by a 7-day break. (Avoid making a common mistake here, which is to start each new packet like the first on the fifth day of the period. This can cause a pregnancy, if the 'period' happens to come on late.)

The snag of this system, or in fact of ever starting later than day 4, is that some women frequently and others quite unexpectedly can have short menstrual cycles. There is then the risk that there may already be a follicle ripening. This could be producing so much natural oestrogen that the pill may be unable to stop the surge of LH hormone from the pituitary which leads to release of an egg (see page 46 and Figures 5 and 6). And so it is always recommended that until the seventh pill of the first course has been taken you should use an effective alternative method of family planning as well, such as the sheath. Obviously it is a bit of a nuisance to be unable to rely on the pill straight away.

Starting on the first day of the period—now the routine

If, in the first cycle only of pill-taking, you start the tablets on the very first day of the period, egg-release is effectively prevented even among women with short cycles. Thus no extra method of family planning need be used. The only problem is that in the first pill cycle this method does seem to cause a bit more 'breakthrough bleeding', which is bleeding on days when you are taking tablets. A part of this is only to be expected, during the first few days, when you are deliberately taking pills during the bleeding of the first period. Another important point to realize is that your first hormone withdrawal bleed on the pill will come on sooner than usual. This is because you will be taking your twenty-first tablet only 21 days after the start of the previous period. As usual on the pill your 'period'/hormone withdrawal bleeding will usually follow only a day or two after that. Thus the very first pill cycle will tend to be only about 23 days long, but this matters not at all. The next packet is started as usual after seven days whether or not a 'period' happens and however long it lasts (see Figure 10).

Notice, by the way, in Figure 10 that the woman had a bit of 'breakthrough' bleeding and spotting, other than at 'period' times. But this minor problem cleared up by the time the third packet of pills was started. This is what usually happens. See pages 73–4 for more about this.

Starting the pill without extra contraceptive precautions is permissible up to day 4 of the cycle. This can be useful sometimes (see page 79). If started any later than day 4 the pill should not be relied on for seven days.

Starting after a recent pregnancy

There is no need to wait for your first period after a baby. Indeed to do so may well mean you 'hit the jackpot' with the very first egg you release after the previous birth, and do not therefore see another period till the next babe arrives! Even if you do not breast-feed, egg-release has never been proved to happen earlier than about four weeks after delivery. So, if bottle-feeding, the Family Planning Association recommends that you should start taking the pill *from the twenty-first day*

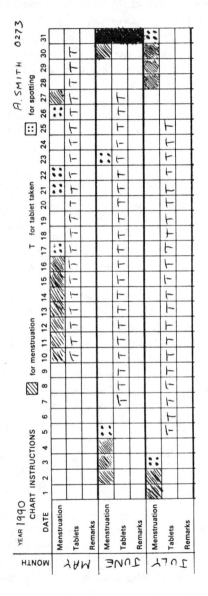

Fig. 10 Diary card—first day start of the pill

after the birth. Twenty-one days later when you finish the first packet you should see the first withdrawal bleed. It is better not to start earlier as this might increase the small risk there is, after any birth, of thrombosis (clotting) in a vein of the legs.

If you are *fully breast-feeding* and plan to continue, then the progestogen-only pill is preferable to the ordinary combined pill. This pill is also started on about *the twenty-first day* following delivery. See Chapter 8 for all you need to know about this very different kind of pill.

After a *suction termination* of pregnancy, or a *spontaneous miscarriage* which has been treated in hospital by a D & C (see Glossary): the pill can be started at once, on the very day of the procedure—or the next day if you are feeling a bit sick. Starting like this immediately protects you against pregnancy, and will mean that, as shown in Figure 10, the first period will occur rather soon—after about 23 days.

If you get unexpected bleeding, as heavy as a period, especially if it is painful, in the first weeks after any early pregnancy has ended, you should *not* call this 'breakthrough' bleeding of the type shown in Figure 10. It could mean that you need a second D & C as the uterus was not emptied out completely. So see your doctor or one of the doctors at the hospital *without delay*.

Why regular pill-taking is so important

If the pill is the method for you, try to take it at about the same time of day. It can be taken morning, noon, or night as long as it is at a roughly constant time, preferably within an hour or two. There is actually a maximum of 12 hours leeway for pregnancy prevention, allowing you to catch up if you forget overnight for example, but it is decidedly 'dodgy' to make a habit of so doing. The reason for being consistent is that after each pill is absorbed, your liver and kidneys, working in combination, are continually eliminating the hormones of the pill from your body. So a gap of more than the usual 24 hours certainly increases the chance of annoying breakthrough bleeding due to too little pill-support to the womb's lining, and *might* even lead to 'breakthrough' egg-release and pregnancy.

This is even more likely if you are late in starting your next packet (i.e. late with the first pill), so prolonging the time when your body has anyway just had a week's rest from the pill's effects (see Figure 11a, page 60). The risk of pregnancy if pills are forgotten is also greater:

(a) if you are on one of the modern ultra-low-dose combined pills shown in Table 9 (page 186). These are very reliable, but have a reduced margin for error;

(b) if you are being treated with any drug which might interfere with the pill's actions, listed on page 70;

(c) possibly also if you have noticed recent 'breakthrough' bleeding (see page 72).

Fortunately, the extra contraceptive actions described in Table 2 (page 46) should still protect you from pregnancy, especially if you obey the rules which follow.

Circumstances which may reduce protection against pregnancy

Missed pills

Do not panic if you forget to take a pill. This is one of the commonest worries that any pill-user ever has. It is unlikely that you will become pregnant. However, it is certainly not something to make a habit of, and most pregnancies on the pill are caused this way. To be as safe as can be you need to follow some simple recommendations. THESE HAVE CHANGED SINCE THE LAST EDITION of this book; the new advice has been agreed by the International Planned Parenthood Federation (IPPF). Extra precautions are advised for less time than the previous (14-day) rule but this is equally valid scientifically—and works! You will find it helpful to keep referring to Figures 11a and 11b.

If you have remembered within less than 12 hours, all you need to do is to take the forgotten pill immediately and then return to your daily routine, taking your next pill at the usual time, even if this means taking two on the same day.

If the delay is more than 12 hours take the omitted pill and the next one at the usual time, even if this means taking two on the same day or at the same time. If more than one pill has been missed, take the latest *missed tablet and the next one on time (or two at once). Get back to regular pill-taking as before* BUT*: Consider yourself not protected for the next seven days, and either abstain from sex or use extra precautions e.g. a method like the condom.*

IF, AND ONLY IF, *you find you have missed one or more of the last seven tablets in the packet (active pills number 15–21 inclusive)* THROW OUT THE REST OF THAT PILL PACK! *Start with pill number one of a new pack* THAT SAME DAY, *leaving no gap between packets just this month. If you are on one of the everyday (ED) brands, miss out the seven inactive 'reminder' pills. (As before, use a back-up method like the condom for seven days).*

This advice for pills missed in the third week means you may not have a period until the end of two packs in a row, but this does you no harm. Nor does it matter, whenever pills have been missed, if for a while you see some 'breakthrough' bleeding on tablet-taking days.

What are extra precautions? Whenever another method is mentioned and any type of pill has recently been or is being taken, this must never be the rhythm, temperature, or cervical mucus methods. The pill's hormones make these quite unusable. Family planners do not recommend spermicides used alone either, and the intra-uterine device (IUD) or coil is unlikely to be useful for so short a time. So what is really meant is either abstinence or a barrier method such as the sheath or one of the types of cap such as the diaphragm used with a spermicide.

The advice here and in Figure 11b may differ from what you read in the leaflet with your packet of pills: beware, sometimes that advice (page 65) is actually unsafe! However, the instructions in all British FPA leaflets since 1989 are very similar and can be used instead. (The only minor difference is explained on page 63.)

What is the justification for this '7-day [plus]' advice? The main point is that any contraceptive is most effective when it is actually being taken, and bound to be least effective when it is not being taken! The pill is a pretty strange contraceptive in that women are told not to take it for a whole week at a time! (See Figure 11a.) This 'lets the body off the hook' so to speak. Though a week is too short a time to allow egg-release, in some

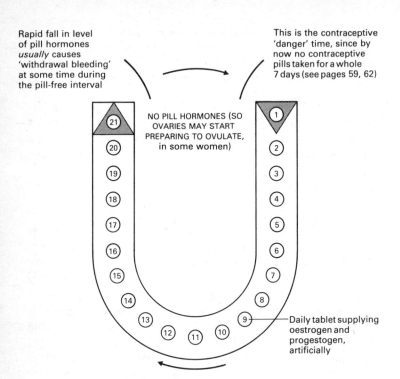

Rapid fall in level of pill hormones *usually* causes 'withdrawal bleeding' at some time during the pill-free interval

This is the contraceptive 'danger' time, since by now no contraceptive pills taken for a whole 7 days (see pages 59, 62)

NO PILL HORMONES (SO OVARIES MAY START PREPARING TO OVULATE, in some women)

㉑ ⑳ ⑲ ⑱ ⑰ ⑯ ⑮ ⑭ ⑬ ⑫ ⑪ ⑩ ⑨ ⑧ ⑦ ⑥ ⑤ ④ ③ ② ①

Daily tablet supplying oestrogen and progestogen, artificially

Fig. IIa The pill cycle (21-day system)

Note: Compare with Figure 7a (page 36). The normal cycle shown there is taken right away and *replaced* by this simpler one. The bleeding from the uterus is caused just by withdrawal of the pill hormones.

Pill-taking is drawn in a horseshoe for the important reason that *a horseshoe is a symmetrical object*. Hence the pill-free interval can be lengthened, leading to the risk of conception, either side of the horseshoe: by forgetting pills either at the beginning *or* at the end of the packet. See text, pages 58–66.

women anything more is too much. So the advice has to cater for the most 'dangerous' tablets to miss, which are those which will lengthen the pill-free time: at the start or finish of a packet, in fact.

AS USUAL, feel free to miss out the more complicated paragraphs which follow, marked with an asterisk (*).

* In all women the menstrual cycle is taken away during the 21 days of pill-taking. Indeed research shows that *once seven*

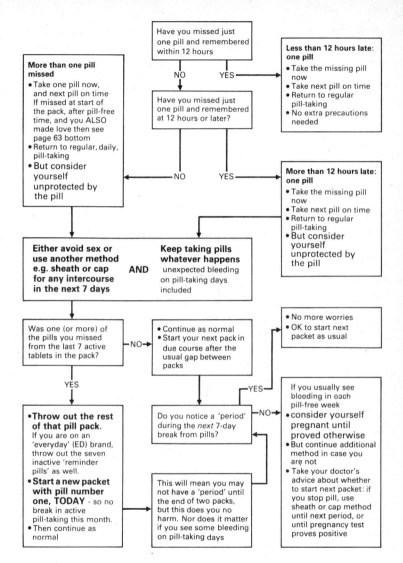

Fig. 11b What to do when pills are taken late or missed altogether

† Or beyond the active pills into the 'dummy' ones if you are on an ED brand (page 52)? If so skip all the dummies just for this month. For progestogen-only pill see Figure 21 (pages 212–13).

tablets have been taken the ovaries are inactive, or 'asleep'. BUT during the pill-free week we have demonstrated at the Margaret Pyke Centre that the blood levels of FSH (from the pituitary gland) and oestrogen (from a growing follicle in one of the ovaries) tend to rise. In some women the rise is more marked than others. If you understand pages 38–42 of the last chapter you will realize this means that the pituitary and ovaries of these women are, if you like, struggling to get free from the suppressing effect of the pill. Any lengthening of the pill-free time beyond seven days means a risk that the ovary 'wakes up': if so the level of oestrogen, in a few women at least, gets to a high enough level to cause a 'surge' of LH and hence egg-release from the largest follicle (see page 40). And egg-release means the risk of pregnancy.

IN SUMMARY:

SEVEN DAYS OF PILL-TAKING PUTS THE OVARIES TO SLEEP.

MORE THAN SEVEN DAYS SINCE PILL-TAKING MIGHT WAKE THE OVARIES UP.

SEVEN DAYS OF NO PILLS IS 'SAFE' (JUST).

How could the pill-free time be lengthened?

First, *forgetting one or more pills at the beginning of a packet*. In fact these are about the most important of all pills to remember to take. Going away for a weekend or longer without one's pills and hence starting the next packet late is a well-known cause of unplanned pregnancy. It is one reason why I personally favour the more widespread use of 28-day (everyday) pill packaging as described on page 52. (A woman who is used to taking pills all the time is likely to have a packet with her wherever she goes.)

The rule should protect a woman who completely misses a pill early in a packet. She must not rely solely on the pill method for seven days from the moment she discovers the problem. This is the time of greatest pregnancy risk, and there is no need to continue with precautions to the end of the packet (as used to be advised), if this means more than seven days.

If two or more tablets were missed very early in a packet, see below (page 64).

How else might the pill-free time be lengthened?

Another way would be by *missing pills at the end of the previous packet*, and then still taking the usual 7-day break.

* In this case the dangerous time for conceiving would not be when the pills were forgotten, but over a week later when— once again—the pituitary and ovary have been 'let off the hook' for longer than usual. In fact pregnancy could result from intercourse during or after the (falsely reassuring) 'period' which comes *after* the missed pills! (This is because that bleeding is not truly a period (pages 47–8), being caused only by the earlier withdrawal of the artificial hormones. It has no connection with what is happening at the ovary.) The egg could be released around the end of the pill-free time *whenever it has been made longer than a week—unless you act . . .*

How should you act? The rule says 'IF, AND ONLY IF, you find you have missed one or more pills in the third week of the packet (active pills number 15–21 inclusive) . . . start with pill number one of a new pack THAT SAME DAY, leaving no gap between packets just this month.' This advice really amounts to '*you made your own break from pill-taking this month, prematurely*, so it would be crazy to add the routine 7-day break on top'.

* Just for interest: you may perhaps notice this is slightly different from the FPA's instruction for Day 15 to 21 pill omissions, in which the current packet would be finished first before proceeding straight to the next one. The main reason is to attempt international agreement in what has been a very muddled area for years. Also the new recommendation is simpler for women taking 'everyday' brands (page 52), who have been known to get muddled about missing out their dummy 'reminder' pills. They now only have to be really clear about which is their Day 1 pill.

What about missing pills in the middle of a packet?

Contrary to what most pill-takers—and some doctors—think, this is *the least dangerous time* to miss tablets, even several in a row. If you follow the argument here, you will see that egg-release and pregnancy are very unlikely because the pills are missed after the pituitary and ovary have been 'put to sleep' by that 'magic minimum' of seven days of pill-taking. It is still better not to be more than 12 hours late even with one pill, though, because of the risk of causing the annoying symptom of 'breakthrough' bleeding (see below). And it is still advised for consistency that you use another method as well for just seven days.

Are the rules different for triphasic pills? No.

* If you have missed pills at the end of a packet and therefore must switch straight to the very low dose of the first phase (see page 192), you are more likely to get a bleed than on a monophasic pill. But with either type the advice does warn about the possibility of bleeding, anyway. *If postponing bleeding more than restoring contraception is your main concern*, and a phasic pill is involved see page 195.

What if I have been so disorganized that I forgot a succession of pills? Should I ask for emergency (post-coital) contraception?

To take a handful of pills will simply make you sick! With one exception (below) it is now recommended that you just take the last missed pill and the next one on time, or both at once if the next is due. You should push out and discard any other forgotten pills. This will ensure that the next tablet, which should follow at the next regular time, will correspond with the correct day of the week as marked on your packet. *Use another method plus the pill for the next seven days (plus if any missed tablet was from the last seven active ones, follow on that same day to the start pill of a new packet).*

The exception is the worst situation, where two or more pills were missed during the first five days of a pack, so effectively lengthening the interval to beyond a week without the pill's contraceptive actions, and you also made love while not taking pills. If, and only if, this applies: ask your doctor for *post-coital hormone treatment* as described on pages 78–9. Return on the next day to regular pill-taking, but be very sure to attend for the planned follow-up examination about four weeks later.

NB post-coital hormones are completely unnecessary if pills are missed at any other time, i.e. in the middle or at the end of a packet. This is because of that slogan 'seven pills are enough to put the ovaries to sleep, and it requires seven pills to be missed to risk waking them up.'

What is the current view of the '14-day rule' of previous editions of 'The Pill'?

This is still a valid alternative. The advice was as follows, if pills were missed:

If the delay is more than 12 hours take the omitted pill and the next one at the usual time, even if this means taking two on the same day.

Then complete the course followed by the 7-day break as usual: but consider yourself no longer sufficiently protected by the pill for the next 14 days.

In other words, for the next 14 days use another effective method as well as the pill whatever happens, continuing if need be during the early days of pill-taking from the next packet.

Disregard for this purpose any bleeding that occurs. If it is the unexpected 'breakthrough' type on pill-taking days, keep taking the pills. *If it is your expected bleeding during the pill-free week, keep on using the other method—unless and until the 14 days are up.*

* This advice 'works' of course because, out of the 14 days' extra precautions, the *second seven days* cover the dangerous time at the end of any pill-free interval which the woman made longer by pills missing at the end of the *previous* pack.

* The 14-day rule is liked by some because it is so simple to explain, and works for 'everyday' pills and in countries where illiteracy is common.

NB there is one rule which is completely WRONG, and that is the one you will still see in many package leaflets: to 'take precautions till the end of the current packet'.

What else may happen if pills are omitted?

Even if egg-release does not occur as a result of missed pills, you are also now more likely to get the problem of 'breakthrough' bleeding.

This is a spotting or sometimes a rather heavier loss, coming on at any time other than the pill-free week. It happens for the same reason as the normal pill 'period': too little at that time of the pill's hormones reaching the lining of the uterus. However, it will almost always stop if you simply disregard it and take pills regularly from now on, using the usual 21 days on, seven days off routine.

What if my next 'period' does not come on? In brief, take advice from your doctor, but continue using some other safe method of family planning like the sheath. This is advisable because absent withdrawal bleeding is only rarely due to pregnancy (see page 49). It would be a pity to become unnecessarily pregnant because you thought you already were, so to speak! Taking the pill will not stop the pregnancy test becoming positive. If new symptoms like nausea, or having to pass urine very frequently, occur—even if you have taken your pills regularly, in fact—you should see your doctor in case they might be due to pregnancy. Take with you for testing a small amount of your first urine of the day in a clean container.

Taking the pill in early pregnancy has not been proved to harm babies (page 129). All the same if you do strongly suspect that you might be pregnant as a result of a pill-taking muddle, most doctors recommend that you transfer to using something like the sheath method, carefully, until you know one way or another. This would also normally be the best policy if for any reason you were unable to discuss the matter with a doctor.

But if you have absolutely *no* reason to suspect reduced protection, then it is in my view best to start the next packet even if there is no bleeding in a particular pill-free week. It would be necessary to see your doctor and arrange a pregnancy test if you began getting the symptoms of pregnancy, or if you went on to miss a second period. See also page 202.

Stomach upsets

From the body's point of view these mean the same as forgetting to take the pills, so the risk of 'breakthrough' egg-release and of 'breakthrough' bleeding are increased in just the same way. The rules to be followed here are shown in Figure

12. If any single episode of *vomiting* was more than three hours after pill-taking, no action is required at all, as by then the pill will have passed beyond your stomach. However, if you vomit back a correctly timed pill after less than three hours you should take another as soon as you feel you will keep it down. If that one stays down and was taken within 12 hours then you can continue to rely on the pill as your method.

The extra pill should ideally be taken from a separate packet or (in emergency) from the end of the current packet, so that you continue taking the right pill for each day of the week. If using a phasic pill (page 192), ensure that the replacement is from the same section of the spare packet. Should your stomach also reject the second pill, you should get back to taking pills as soon as you are able to keep them down. IF *the vomiting involved tablets from the last seven active ones in a packet, go straight to the start pill of a new pack. In addition* you should consider yourself no longer protected. Use an extra method such as the sheath or cap plus a spermicide during however long the stomach upset itself lasts, plus for seven days from when it ends.

Diarrhoea if alone (no vomiting) has to be 'of cholera-like proportions' to interfere with the absorption of the pill. If it *is* like that, which means like water and every few minutes, follow the advice just given for a bad attack of vomiting. Otherwise just keep taking your tablets. (*Note the advice here has again changed since previous editions*.)

See also page 66 for what to do if you fail to see the next 'period'.

Taking other medicines along with the pill

To be effective, the pill must be absorbed, be transported in the blood, perform its actions, and then be eliminated from the body. A number of other drugs can apparently interfere with some of these complex processes. Such interference (interaction) can lower the blood levels of the pill hormones and so lead to the risk of egg-release and therefore pregnancy. See Table 3.

* This weakening contraception effect can be caused in various ways. *Enzyme inducers* are drugs which in addition to their main effect have a simulating action on the special liver

● Vomiting

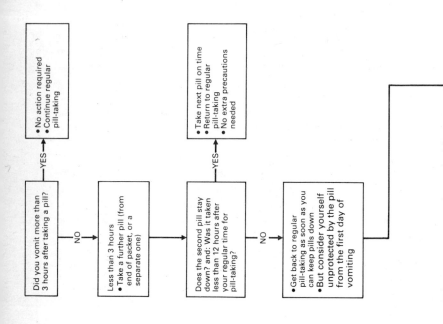

Did you vomit more than 3 hours after taking a pill?

YES → ● No action required ● Continue regular pill-taking

NO ↓

Less than 3 hours
● Take a further pill (from end of packet, or a separate one)

→ Does the second pill stay down? and: Was it taken less than 12 hours after your regular time for pill-taking?

YES → ● Take next pill on time ● Return to regular pill-taking ● No extra precautions needed

NO ↓

● Get back to regular pill-taking as soon as you can keep pills down ● But consider yourself unprotected by the pill from the first day of vomiting

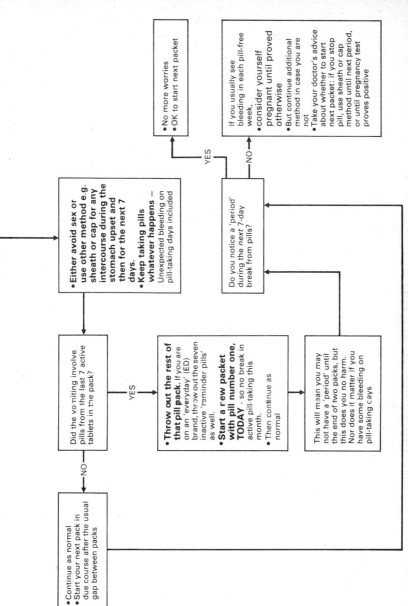

Fig. 12 What to do in the event of a stomach upset

Flowchart content:

- Either avoid sex or use other method e.g. sheath or cap for any intercourse during the stomach upset and then for the next 7 days.
- Keep taking pills whatever happens – Unexpected bleeding on pill-taking days included

Did the vomiting involve pills from the last 7 active tablets in the pack?

NO →
- Continue as normal
- Start your next pack in due course after the usual gap between packs

YES →
- **Throw out the rest of that pill pack.** If you are on an 'everyday' (ED) brand, throw out the seven inactive 'reminder pills' as well.
- **Start a new packet with pill number one, TODAY** - so no break in active pill-taking this month.
- Then continue as normal

This will mean you may not have a 'period' until the end of two packs, but this does you no harm. Nor does it matter if you have some bleeding on pill-taking days

Do you notice a 'period' during the next 7-day break from pills?

YES →
- No more worries
- OK to start next packet

NO →
If you usually see bleeding in each pill-free week,
- consider yourself pregnant until proved otherwise
- But continue additional method in case you are not
- Take your doctor's advice about whether to start next packet: if you stop pill, use sheath or cap method until next period, or until pregnancy test proves positive

The pill: how do I take it? 69

***Table 3** Drugs which are suspected of interfering with the pill, to cause 'breakthrough' bleeding and increased risk of pregnancy. Evidence for this is stronger for some drugs on this list (in *italic*) than for others. Common brand names are in brackets

---

Drugs to treat epilepsy

phenobarbitone (Luminal)
   and other barbiturates
phenytoin (Epanutin)

primidone (Mysoline)
carbamazepine (Tegretol)

The only drugs for epilepsy that do not interfere at all appear to be sodium valproate (Epilim) and clonazepam (Rivotril). But these are not necessarily the right choice.

Sedatives and tranquillizers

meprobamate (Equanil)

Drugs to treat infections

rifampicin (Rimactane)—used in the treatment of *tuberculosis*

Many other antibiotics, such as *amoxycillin (Amoxyl)* and *tetracyclines*, are also under suspicion of interfering with the combined pill only, not POP—but see note below.

Miscellaneous drugs

spironolactone (Aldactone)
griseofulvin (Grisovin)

phenylbutazone (Butazolidin)
dichloralphenazone (Welldorm)

Cigarette smoke

There is new evidence, not fully confirmed, that smoking *may* reduce the pill's contraceptive effects.

Note: **This is *not* a complete list.** Other drug interactions remain to be clarified. Several have been deliberately omitted here because so far there is too little evidence that, in practice, they cause any problem for pill-users. *Co-trimoxazole (Septrin)*, certainly, and metronidazole (Flagyl), possibly, actually enhance the pill's effects by inhibiting the liver's actions. Compare with Vitamin C (page 92), which strengthens the effect of oestrogen in a different way.

enzymes which normally inactivate the hormones before they are disposed of in the bowels and in the urine. So more inactivation means weaker contraception. In a very few women (no one knows which, so it is safest to assume all might be affected) so-called *broad spectrum antibiotics* might stop the special system which keeps up the levels of oestrogen by reabsorbing some which escapes to the gut from the liver. (This antibiotic effect does not affect progestogen and therefore causes no problem for users of the POP—page 214.)

Implications. In general, the golden rules are obviously:

(a) to tell the person who prescribes you the pill about all other drugs you are taking, and

(b) to inform any other doctor about to prescribe you *any drug* that you use the pill.

For safety, ask specifically if a drug might affect the pill . . .

1. *Short-term treatment* (less than a month). If you are put on a relevant medicine, especially one from Table 3—but not all are listed—use another method such as the sheath throughout the treatment, and *when it finishes start the main 7-day 'rule' as for vomiting* (above, page 67 and Figure 12).

2. *Long-term treatment* (over a month).

(a) *Relevant antibiotics (not rifampicin or griseofulvin).* The special oestrogen-raising system mentioned above depends on friendly bacteria in the gut which are killed by the antibiotic. These become resistant to the antibiotic after about four weeks, and so they come back in good enough numbers to do their good work. This is why extra precautions are unnecessary if you are already on long-term low-dose tetracycline for acne when starting the pill. The only time they are needed is during the first four weeks of antibiotic treatment if started in a current pill-taker. Extra oestrogen (perhaps by using a pill from Table 10, page 188) is an alternative way of reducing this small and short-term pregnancy risk—and improves acne! See page 204.

(b) *Enzyme inducers, used long term.* The drugs concerned are chiefly treatments for tuberculosis or epilepsy, see Table 3. First, these patients need to consider using another method of contraception altogether. After discussion though, many can continue to use the pill under careful medical supervision.

They should naturally use a slightly higher-dose pill, from the list in Table 10 (page 188), to compensate for the lowered blood levels caused by the enzyme inducer. This is still a low-dose pill for them, of course—it is a bit like climbing up a 'down' escalator to stay in the same place. Following the reasoning on pages 58–63, my advice is that they also take fewer potentially 'dangerous' breaks than usual between pill packets (i.e. they use the tricycling scheme, page 52); and the break after each run of three packets is additionally shortened to five days.

Watch for 'breakthrough' bleeding (see page 200 for more details). Even if the other drug you are taking, perhaps one you bought yourself at the chemist, is not on the list in Table 3—but particularly if it is—watch out for bleeding on tablet-taking days. This so-called 'breakthrough' bleeding coming on for the first time after starting another drug can be *the early warning sign of too low a blood level of the pill's hormones*. It should always make you discuss the matter promptly with whoever prescribes you the pill. A stronger one may be required.

Effect of the pill on other drugs

The opposite kind of interference is also possible, in which the pill alters the action of another drug. Fortunately very few instances of this actually make any important difference to treatment. Again, the main thing from your point of view is, *if in doubt, ask* if the other drug matters at all, either way.

This whole problem of drugs interfering with each other highlights the tendency these days to take too many medicines of all kinds, maybe sometimes without a very good reason.

Change of pills from a higher- to a lower- or ultra-low-dose variety

This matter of the different brands of pills will make more sense when you have read Chapter 7. However, the question of changing to a lower-dose pill needs to be considered here, as this is another time when there could be some loss of contraceptive protection. At the change-over time the steady suppression by the pill of the woman's natural hormones from her pituitary and ovary is reduced, just enough perhaps to allow 'breakthrough' egg-release 'on the rebound'. However, once she is safely established on the new ultra-low-dose pill, she is effectively protected against pregnancy. The extra pregnancy risk is only at the time of the change-over and is small. It can be virtually eliminated by taking extra precautions while taking the first seven pills if there is the usual gap between packets. Or, more simply, the recommended method is to *start the new lower-dose variety the very next day after finishing the current higher-dose packet*. Pills are then taken daily for 21 days, followed by a 7-day break as usual.

If you follow this system you may have bleeding like a pill 'period' during the first seven days of tablet-taking from your new low-dose packet. Or you may have no bleeding at all till after the end of that new packet. Either is quite normal, and your protection against pregnancy is maintained throughout.

This problem never of course arises when moving to a definitely higher-dose pill, which can be done after the usual 7-day break. If you are ever left in doubt about what your new pill is, act as though it is lower dose.

For the rules about changing from a combined (ordinary) pill to a progestogen-only variety or back again, see Chapter 8.

Side-effects

These are all going to be considered fully later, but a few general points need making here in this practical chapter about pill-taking.

Side-effects are effects extra to the main actions of any drug, which in the case of the pill are those shown in Table 2 (page 46). They can be good or bad, and the good ones are much too often forgotten. The effects which are unwanted fall into two main types: *uncommon side-effects*, some of which can be serious; and *commoner* ones which are almost never serious but do cause enough nuisance or trouble to make some people change to a different pill or perhaps a different method.

Considering the commoner ones first, they can be divided into two further groups as follows:

1. *Side-effects related to the bleeding pattern*
- *'Breakthrough' bleeding and spotting* (bleeding or spotting on tablet-taking days)
- *Absence of pill 'periods'* (no bleeding on the tablet-free days)

See pages 66, 200–1.

Except on the advice of your doctor, *neither* problem should be allowed to affect your daily pill-taking routine. Let the pill packet rule your pill-taking, not the bleeding pattern—whatever that may be. Do not stop taking pills before the end of a packet because of bleeding even if it seems like a period. Pregnancies have happened that way . . . Just keep taking successive packets and wait for the arrival of the normal bleeding pattern in due course. If in doubt, see your doctor: especially if reduced protection is a possibility (pages 58–72 and also 200–1).

More details about how these problems can be handled are given in Chapter 7 along with a helpful diagram (Figure 20, pages 200–1).

2. *Other minor side-effects (so-called*: they often do not seem so). These include nausea, headaches, breast tenderness or tingling, gain in weight, vaginal discharge, leg aches and cramps, mild depression, and loss of interest in sex. All these and more have been reported by pill-users, but don't cross bridges. You may well have no side-effects at all and could even feel extra well while taking the pill. This is much more commonly so now that the dose given has been so much reduced. However, every woman reacts in her own special way, and the first pill tried is not always the best for you. As there are more than 20 varieties of pill, if you do have problems it is usually possible to find a different brand that suits you better. This is all fully discussed using the idea of 'pill-ladders' in Chapter 7 (Figures 17–20, pages 185–204).

A very important point to remember is to give any particular brand a good try before giving up, and this usually means using it for at least three months. If either bleeding or other-type minor side-effects occur, they usually do settle down after the first two or three courses of pills. If you look again at the list above, several of the symptoms, such as nausea, breast tenderness, and gain in weight, also happen in the first few months of pregnancy. This is partly because the pill imitates pregnancy in some ways, but it is probably just a coincidence that, as in pregnancy, the symptoms usually improve after the third month!

More major or serious side-effects

These are also discussed in much more detail later. For completeness I am including here a list of those symptoms which, though most unlikely to occur, should lead you to contact a doctor at once and to inform him or her that you are taking the pill. They may or may not mean anything serious or even be anything to do with the pill. *But they do mean that you should*

(a) *stop the pill until further notice* (but transfer to using another effective method)

(b) *come under medical care without delay*

so the diagnosis can be made and the right treatment started.

1. Severe pain in the calf of one leg, especially if linked with swelling (not the aching legs that so many people get, nor simple painless swelling of both ankles).

2. Severe central pain in the chest. Severe sharp pains in either side of the chest, aggravated by breathing.

3. Unexplained breathlessness, or cough with blood-stained phlegm.

4. Severe pain in the abdomen.

5. Any unusually severe, prolonged headache, particularly if of migraine type, especially if it is the first ever such attack or gets worse with the passage of time or keeps returning (page 101).

6. A bad fainting attack, or first ever epileptic fit.

7. Sudden weakness, or very *marked* numbness and tingling *suddenly* affecting one side or one part of the body. NB This is not to be confused with the carpal tunnel syndrome, page 136.

8. Sudden loss of part of the field of vision.

9. Sudden disturbance of the ability to speak normally.

10. A severe and generalized, perhaps painful, skin rash (page 135).

11. Jaundice (yellow eyes and skin).

12. Very high blood pressure (page 172).

Number 12 is something which can be diagnosed by a doctor or nurse only when routinely measuring the blood pressure. Also jaundice may well first be noticed by a doctor or other observer.

I must stress again that most women can take the pill for years and years without getting a single one of these frightening symptoms. They are also practically the only reasons important enough for the pill to be stopped at once, in the middle of a packet. Otherwise make a routine appointment to see your doctor and continue to the end of a packet. This reduces the chance of an unplanned pregnancy (and erratic bleeding). In fact, if the doctor is able to reassure you that your symptom from the list above is not due to anything serious and is *not* due to the pill, you can of course restart pill-taking, following the rules of Figure 11.

Two other reasons for stopping the pill

1. *Immobilization.* This means being confined to bed, as might occur rather suddenly, for instance after an accident. It is recommended that you tell the doctor and stop the pill at once. Being kept in bed makes blood clotting in the veins of the leg more probable, and the pill may increase that risk. See also page 174.

2. *Major operations.* The chances of a blood clot in deep veins of the legs are increased by the operation itself, as well as by the confinement to bed which obviously follows it. Being on the pill will of course never stop you having an emergency, life-saving operation such as for appendicitis—but you must inform the surgeon. Heparin (blood-thinning) treatment may be required. It is better when you have the chance to stop the pill at least four weeks before a planned major operation, such as gallstone surgery.

See page 174 for more details.

Unless your gynaecologist tells you otherwise, it is usually perfectly in order for you to continue on the pill right up to the time of a female sterilization procedure—which is a minor operation—and then just to finish the current packet.

Coming off the pill

There is no need to make any routine breaks from the pill every few months or years in order to preserve your fertility or for any other reason. Secondly, after stopping the pill it is very common for the first spontaneous or natural period to be a bit delayed. But two-thirds of women have their first period by six weeks after their last pill 'period', and by six months nearly all have got back their own periods. So a 'wait and see' policy is best. If this, or anything else, is a worry to you do not hesitate to discuss it with your family doctor or with the clinic doctor who prescribes you the pill. Actually, many women find out the hard way that their fertility is in fine shape after stopping the pill: by getting pregnant so very easily that they cannot believe it! So if you are not ready for a baby, be warned and consider staying on the pill or use another safe method from the day you stop. NB *not the rhythm method*—this is totally unreliable just after a course of pills. See pages 250–6.

If you go overdue after stopping the pill you may be worried that your new method of family planning has let you down. In that case wait until it is at least five weeks since your last pill 'period', which is four weeks from the earliest likely egg-release. Then arrange a pregnancy test on a small amount of your first urine of the day. Commonly it will be negative and remain so if repeated, until you see your first natural period in due course.

Very occasionally the first period is very much delayed, and if so it is sensible to take medical advice: but not until six months have gone by. A few tests are essential, to check that your pituitary gland and ovaries are in good working order, though currently 'resting'. But usually nothing more needs to be done to bring back your menstrual cycle, with the usual release of eggs and periods: until, that is, you wish to try for a baby. See page 181 for more re absence of periods.

Stopping the pill to have a baby

Obstetricians usually prefer that women who stop the pill for this reason use another contraceptive method, such as the sheath or the diaphragm, until they have seen at least one natural period—which means one later than the bleeding which followed a few days after the last packet of pills. This helps them to calculate the date the baby is due, though this is much less important now with routine use of ultrasound scanning. Some experts recommend that *ideally* you should wait for two natural periods before trying for a baby. See pages 127–8. There is no proof that this is beneficial, though it can do no harm.

Emergency contraception/post-coital contraception

This has often been called the 'morning after pill', but there is a battle on at present to try to eliminate that misleading name. This is because it is possible to use hormone treatment to prevent pregnancy, starting *much later* than the next morning after unprotected intercourse—*up to 72 hours* later in fact. Accidents do happen—sheaths rupturing or slipping off, for instance; not to mention rape. In my view there are therefore definitely some cases for whom this treatment is appropriate. It is believed often to act by preventing implantation (page 37), so it is not causing an abortion. Others may disagree: see pages 235–6 for discussion of some ethical aspects.

Nowadays the usual hormone treatment is two tablets of a particular 50 mcg oestrogen-containing pill, taken in the doctor's surgery or clinic, followed by two more exactly 12 hours later. You will notice that I do not name the pill brand(s) used. This is deliberate. Readers should resist the temptation to 'dabble' in this kind of treatment, without medical supervision.

Why a doctor should be involved

Correct use of the correct pills is important. A vaginal examination and blood pressure check should be done before treatment and often also subsequent to the next period. Side-effects occur, chiefly nausea, sometimes vomiting. Even the decision to treat at all is not that simple. The chances of conception can sometimes be judged by the doctor to be so low that the risks of treatment are greater than those of just waiting for the next period. The other method of treatment, with an IUD (page 233) put in up to five days after ovulation, may occasionally be medically preferable: for instance because of its greater effectiveness, or because the hormone method works much less well beyond 72 hours after intercourse, or if other risks were also taken earlier in the cycle. If there is already a pregnancy the hormone treatment will not cause an abortion. The method can fail, in about two in 100 cases treated overall, more if the risk was taken around ovulation. And the possibility of a pregnancy being harmed by the hormones cannot be ruled out: though the risk at such an early time, before implantation (page 37) is thought to be *even less* than the low estimate on page 130. Very rarely, an ectopic pregnancy can occur (page 218). Also, see pages 64, 214 for some special treatment situations.

All in all this 'morning after' treatment is not that simple and should be used only in emergency, not repeatedly as a method of birth control. The need for it should be removed by arranging a recognized method for the future.

As the hormone method can sometimes work by just delaying egg-release, it is vital to use a method like the sheath until the start of the next period anyway. In appropriate cases, insertion of an IUD has the obvious advantage of solving both the immediate and the longer-term family planning problem. Alternatively, it can be removed next month, having dealt with the immediate crisis.

If the hormone method is used and the woman plans to use the pill in future, she should be sure that the next bleeding is truly a period before taking the first tablet. But if she takes it by the *fourth day* she can then rely on the new method, as though she had used the first-day system (page 55). See also page 234.

Above all, every woman having this treatment must be fully counselled and attend for follow-up to ensure it has worked . . .

How to obtain contraceptive advice

Already you may be thinking there seems a lot to take in about the pill. Actually, most advice about ordinary pill-taking can be summed up:

> *continue taking your tablets according to the normal routine regardless of any development—except one of those mentioned on pages 75–6—until you can talk to someone who knows the answers.*

All users of the pill should have access to such a trained person. This is usually a doctor but often a nurse, who can go over the points that apply to you personally.

What happens at the first family planning visit?

The exact procedure will depend quite a lot on where you go to get the pill. It is your right to choose where. Clinics are often chosen by teenagers. You may even go to a different general practitioner from the one who normally sees you for other medical matters. The arrangements vary: between different family doctors' surgeries, between different clinics, and in different countries. *As a minimum* you should always be asked some questions about your medical history in order to establish that you are suitable for the pill. Your age and smoking habits should be noted and you should be weighed and have your blood pressure checked.

In Britain and many other countries the addresses of family planning clinics are to be found in the telephone directory. If you choose to go to one of them, you do not need to bring any doctor's letter with you. Your name is taken first at the reception desk—no objection whatsoever being made if you are unmarried—and your date of birth, address, and similar items are noted. A more confidential set of details is taken by a nurse in a separate side-room. She usually has a standard card to complete and all you have to do is answer her questions. She needs to know if you have had an abortion or miscarriage or ever had treatment for a sexually transmitted disease. The nurse plays a most important role in the modern family planning clinic. It is she who usually checks your weight and blood pressure, and tests your urine if necessary. (Specially trained nurses often do much more, including examinations.)

Then you will be called to see the doctor, everything again being completely confidential. There will normally be no problem about your partner coming in with you, if you would both like that. The doctor describes and discusses the various methods of family planning, and answers your questions about the pill if that is the method you are planning to use. Heart disease (page 97) and cancer (page 138) are important aspects usually discussed now, though if you have no special concerns they may be postponed till a later visit. If there are any special points—for instance, if you are a smoker over 35, or are uneasy and feel ill-informed, or are under or not long past the legal age of consent—then time should be made for a longer discussion on all the pros and cons.

The examination

Contrary to what is believed by many women and by some doctors this is *not* a vital part of the first visit to start on the pill—apart, that is, from taking the blood pressure (which is indeed something you should insist on having done, see page 86). However, it is good preventive medicine to have the breasts examined to be sure there are no lumps, and to learn how to do this regularly yourself; to have a vaginal examination to check that the uterus, uterine tubes, and ovaries are normal; and to have a cervical smear test done. The latter should be done regularly in all sexually active women, especially pill-takers. But if you have not yet started having intercourse, or are anxious about it, there is absolutely no rush for it at this stage. It can often be better done at a later visit.

If you have never had an internal examination, a brief description may be helpful. Women who were afraid of this beforehand usually wonder afterwards what they were worrying about. If you are relaxed it is entirely painless and very quick. In the *bimanual examination* the doctor uses both hands, the left hand on the abdomen and two gloved fingers of the right hand inside the vagina.

The second part of the examination is with an instrument called a *speculum*. This takes up only a little more space in the vagina than the doctor's gloved two fingers did. Some women like to put it in for themselves, so you should be free to ask about that if you wish. The speculum is designed to open out a little so that the walls of the vagina and the entrance to the uterus (the cervix) can be inspected. Using a flat wooden or plastic spatula the doctor may painlessly wipe some loose cells from the cervix on to a glass slide. A tiny 'bottle-brush' called a 'Cytobrush' is now often rotated within the cervix as well. The test may cause some bleeding for a few hours, like the end of a period. All the smear material obtained on the slide is then sent to the laboratory to check that the cells are normal. This is all there is to the well-known cervical smear or 'Pap smear' test. See also pages 28, 142, and 263, Questions 13 and 14.

The speculum is also used if swabs need to be taken and sent to the lab. This could be because you have noticed a big increase in the amount of normal vaginal discharge. With or without this, swabs are often taken if you have complained of soreness or itching or pain on intercourse.

Usually only three months' supply of the chosen pill is given at first. This is to make sure that you return for a further check-up, particularly of your blood pressure and weight, and for further supplies at that time. If you need special medical supervision for any reason, you may be asked to come back sooner.

What if I am under age?

If you are under a certain age (16 in Britain), in many countries your partner will be breaking the law if you have intercourse. Plenty of couples do break this law. But there is a lot more to consider—you might like to read pages 23–31 if you have not already done so, and carefully weigh up the pros and the cons. If you are able to say 'wait' you will save yourself from a lot of worry, and some risks.

On the other hand, if you are already having intercourse under age, know the dangers involved but feel that you will continue, you will find that most doctors nowadays are prepared to prescribe you the pill—without moralizing. If you have not already done so they will strongly encourage you to tell at least one of your parents—the law recommends but does not enforce this and you could be agreeably surprised by their reaction. The doctor might offer to do this for you if you would prefer: but should do so only with your permission, not behind your back.

Doctors are permitted to prescribe you the pill even without the definite consent of your mother or father, if in their medical judgement you are seriously at risk of the even greater problem of an unwanted pregnancy. *You will find the Brook Advisory clinics (see Useful addresses) particularly helpful, as they specialize in providing 100 per cent confidential help for teenagers in all sex and family planning matters.*

German measles (Rubella)

This illness, although it is so mild in the mother, can very seriously damage a developing baby during pregnancy. If you plan to have a baby at any time, it is sensible forward planning while you are safely protected against conceiving to have the simple blood test to show whether you have immunity to Rubella. About one out of every eight women in Britain who has this test done is found to be at risk. Do not rely on a history of German measles in the past: this is often wrong as other infections can imitate it. If you are not immune the vaccination is not painful and it is well worth having. Like the blood test it can easily be arranged by whoever supplies you with the pill. Although it is *believed* not to be harmful, you should not be pregnant when vaccinated and ideally should avoid pregnancy for one month afterwards. Hence the logic of getting this matter sorted out while you are still on the pill or using another effective method.

To conclude, let me stress that family planning clinics simply want to help, in many ways over and above avoiding an unwanted pregnancy. For a start, they are also very ready to help those who are a bit late, and think they might already be pregnant. It is never too late to go to a clinic and talk things through. If the early morning specimen of urine (which you should take with you in a clean glass bottle) shows that you are in fact pregnant, clinics can arrange appropriate counselling about the pregnancy. Most family planning nurses and doctors are easy to talk to, and are very helpful too if you have emotional problems or difficulties with any aspect of sex including becoming pregnant (infertility) or intercourse itself. Special counselling can be arranged for couples where sex has become a problem.

Most of what I have described in the last few pages applies also if you go to your family doctor rather than to a clinic for your pills. The visits may tend to be briefer partly because he or she probably knows most of the important medical facts about you already. It is entirely up to you whether you prefer to go to a clinic or to your doctor's office or surgery. Better organized practices now run at least one special or 'dedicated' family planning session each week. You should get more time there, for discussion, or for the fitting of a cap or IUD.

Follow-up visits

For pill-users the first return visit is commonly after three months, and then blood pressure and weight checks should be done as a routine every 6–12 months. An internal examination will only need to be done when you have the next regular cervical smear, now often taken by the family planning nurse.

Last but not least

Never hesitate to go back to whoever prescribed your pills, immediately perhaps, or certainly sooner than your next routine visit, if you ever have doubts or anxieties about using the pill, or about any effect it seems to having on you.

4

....

The pill: will it make me ill?
Diseases of the circulation

The pregnancy-preventing or contraceptive effects of the pill
were described in Chapter 2. The next two chapters summarize
what we know about its other effects, starting here with changes
in the chemistry of the body, and the very important effects the
pill can have on the blood, heart, arteries, and veins.

We all know that reading any medical book tends to be rather
alarming because we immediately begin to feel that we are
suffering from most of the diseases it describes. Do you tend to
expect the worst all the time? If so, remind yourself how many
millions of women take the pill (page 3) and that the majority
stay entirely well. The list of side-effects which have ever been
linked with the pill is a long one, and the next two chapters are
bound to seem a bit threatening to some people. So be sure not
to stop there but carry on and read Chapter 6, to help you to
see things in proportion. But provided you are not someone
who should avoid the method altogether for medical reasons—
this is discussed in Chapter 7—the chances of your getting any
one of all the complications described here is very small.

Toxicity (poisoning)

One of the very good points about the pill is that unlike so
many drugs on the market, and that includes many such as
aspirin and paracetamol which can actually be bought over the
counter, it seems to be almost impossible to take a fatal or even
dangerous overdose. Let us be clear what this means: it is
certainly possible for particular individuals unexpectedly to be
very seriously harmed even by the normal dose of the pill. What

I am saying here is that the general 'average person'—whether woman or man, or even a young child—is unlikely to be harmed even by taking a large handful of pills. Toddlers have been known to swallow dozens of their mothers' pills and apart from feeling or being rather sick at the time have ended up none the worse for the experience.

If the patient should be a baby girl, after a few days she may well have a 'period'. This is because the hormones have stimulated the lining of her tiny uterus. It therefore grows just as it would do 15 years later in the menstrual cycle, or if she took the pill. Hence, as her body gets rid of the swallowed pill hormones, a harmless hormone withdrawal bleed follows in the usual way. See pages 47–9.

Without emergency treatment, on the other hand, swallowing a similar number of iron or paracetamol (Panadol) tablets might be fatal. But obviously the pill, like all medicines, should be kept secure and out of the reach of children.

*Body chemistry

All the effects to be described later must have their ultimate explanation in the chemistry of the body. So it seems logical to make this our starting-point. More than 100 different laboratory tests on blood, urine, and other body fluids have given abnormal results in women on the pill. See Table 4, which shows just a few of the more important changes which have been described.

Many of the alterations are similar to those that would be found in normal pregnancy. This is not surprising. It was explained in Chapter 2 that, from the body's point of view, being on the pill in many ways mimics being pregnant. The fact that these changes are similar to those in pregnancy is somewhat reassuring. Pregnancy after all is a perfectly 'normal' condition and many women have a whole succession of pregnancies and live long and healthy lives. On the other hand, pregnancy is linked with an increased risk of several conditions including thrombosis which I shall be considering shortly in connection with the pill.

In spite of much research, we have as yet no idea what some

of the changes in body chemistry mean in practice. Quite a number, such as the changes in blood-clotting factors, connected with oestrogen, have an obvious link with one of the known side-effects of the pill. Others which are so far unexplained may in due course be shown to lie behind a known or still unknown unwanted effect, or equally possibly some benefit of the pill. Others could turn out in the end to be entirely neutral changes.

As a general working rule (as proposed by Professor Victor Wynn, of London) to play safe means that '*if we can measure any substance in the pill-user's body, we would like it to be normal—or as near normal as possible*.' So a lot of research is in progress to produce pills with minimal effects on the system. See pages 153–6.

One consequence of the changes in the body chemistry is that whenever you visit a doctor it is most important to remind him of the fact if you are on the pill. This is particularly necessary if some specimen, such as a blood test, is going to be sent to a laboratory. The lab may be unable to interpret the results of the test satisfactorily unless this information is given.

*Effects on the blood levels of sugar and of fats

You will recall that the pill has two hormones, oestrogen and progestogen. The *older high-dose pills* used to cause changes in the ability to deal with the rise in blood sugar that occurs after eating a meal. This is usually tested for by giving the patient a drink containing a measured amount of the most important blood sugar of the body (glucose) and then for up to three hours afterwards taking frequent blood and urine samples. This test is known as the oral Glucose Tolerance Test, and abnormal results like those in people with a very mild form of diabetes were found in some pill-takers.

Then came *pills with a lower dose (less than 50 mcg)* of the oestrogen hormone (better for the thrombosis problem, see below), but they still had what we now consider too high doses of the progestogens—known as norethisterone (NET) and levonorgestrel (LNG). Such pills, in common use during the 1970s and 1980s, tended to raise levels of the hormone insulin, which normally controls the level of blood glucose. See pages 154–5. But none of the studies of these older pills showed that

The pill: will it make me ill?   87

*Table 4 Some changes in body chemistry

	Blood level	Remarks
Liver		
Liver functioning ● *generally*	Altered in all users	These many changes cause no apparent harm to the liver itself, except in the tiny minority who develop jaundice. The liver is *involved*, however, in the production of most of the changes in blood level of substances shown in this table, including the important changes in blood sugar, fats, and clotting factors.
Albumin (*the main protein of blood*)	→ ↓	
Transaminases (*special liver enzymes*)	↑	
Amino acids ('building blocks' for body proteins)	Altered	
Blood sugar (glucose) after a meal	↑	These changes, hardly shown with the latest pills, may partly explain the increased risk of thrombosis in arteries. See page 87.
Blood fats (lipids)	Altered (mostly ↑)	
Clotting factors ● *generally*	mostly ↑	See pages 93–4. Both the pill and smoking affect these interrelated systems, connected with the risk of thrombosis. Fibrinolysis is enhanced in the blood, but *reduced* in the vessel walls.
Anti-thrombin III (special anti-clotting factor)	→	
Fibrinolysis (the system to get rid of blood clots once formed)	↓	
Tendency for platelets to stick to each other (platelet aggregation)	↑	
Hormones		
Insulin	↓	These hormone changes are thought to be connected with those affecting blood sugar and blood lipids (above).
Growth hormone	↓	
Steroid hormones from adrenal gland	↑	
Thyroid gland hormones	↑	See page 90.
Luteinizing hormone (LH)	↓	Lowering the levels of these hormones is essential for the pill's contraceptive actions (see page 45).
Follicle stimulating hormone (FSH)	↓	
Natural oestrogen	↓	
Natural progesterone	↓	
Prolactin	↑	Can cause milky fluid from breasts (see page 131).

Minerals and vitamins

Iron	↑	
Copper	↑	This is a good effect (see page 91).
Zinc	↓	
Vitamins A, K	↑	
Riboflavine, folic acid	↓	Effects unknown, but not believed to cause any
Vitamin B₆ (pyridoxine)	↓	health risk in most pill-users. Pyridoxine is discussed
Vitamin B₁₂ (cyanocobalamin)	↓	on page 108.
Vitamin C (ascorbic acid)	↓	

Binding globulins

Binding globulins	↑	These special substances carry hormones and minerals mostly in an inactive way in the blood. Because their levels increase in parallel with them, the *effective* blood levels of the hormones or minerals are not much altered.

Blood viscosity	↑	
Body water	↑	This retention of fluids explains some of the weight gain blamed on the pill (see page 92).

Factors affecting blood pressure

Renin substrate	Altered	
Renin activity	↑	This is a very complicated story. Changes do not
Angiotensin II	↑	correlate as well as expected with the actual blood
Output of the heart	↑	pressure levels (see page 102).

Immunity/allergy system

Number of white blood cells	↑	
Immunoglobulins (antibodies)		See page 137.
Function of the lymphocytes	Altered	

Note: In the table arrow up ↑ means the level usually goes up, arrow down ↓ means the level tends to go down. 'Altered' means that the changes are known to be more complex, with both increases and decreases occurring in different substances within the system.

the fully developed condition of diabetes occurred. Those few pill-users who developed diabetes, and needed injections of insulin or tablet treatment for it, were thought to be people who would in due course have been affected anyway.

Then during the 1980s came the *ultra-low-dose NET and LNG pills* followed, finally, by pills containing the *latest progestogens desogestrel* (DSG, as in Marvelon and Mercilon) and *gestodene* (GSD, as in Femodene and Minulet)—all of which had negligible effects on glucose or insulin.

The earlier pill types which altered glucose or insulin levels also caused changes to lipids (blood fats), similar to those which have been found in some women (and men) who have an above-average risk of heart attacks and strokes because of disease of their arteries. It is not known whether these changes meant the same when caused by the pill as when observed in studies of general populations. However, the two types of pill described last above—the ultra-low dose and DSG- or GSD-containing ones—have minimal or no adverse effects on the lipids anyway and are now preferred for general use. See pages 155, 189–90.

If even before taking the pill you are known to have one of the rare disorders causing abnormal blood fats—sometimes called hyperlipidaemia, or hypercholesterolaemia—then the *combined* pill should be avoided. A family history of heart attacks or strokes occurring in young near relatives under age 45 is an important clue to this potential problem. If this applies to you discuss the matter with your doctor even if you will not be taking the pill—you may be found to need a special diet or other treatment. See page 172.

* *Effects on the body's own hormones*

Some of the more important changes which have been discovered are listed in Table 4. See the various comments in the Remarks column.

* *The thyroid gland*

Although the total level of thyroid hormones rises in the blood, they are chiefly carried in an inactive way by the special thyroid hormone binding globulin (see Table 4). So their effects on the body are generally not altered. In fact there is now some reason to believe that the pill may actually protect the user against thyroid disease. This beneficial effect of the pill seems to apply to both over-activity and under-activity of the gland.

*Effects on blood levels of minerals and vitamins

The vitamin and mineral changes shown in Table 4 have not been shown to cause any harm at all to most women. They have caused concern to some nutritionists that pill-use might cause symptoms of deficiency diseases in poorly nourished women. However, studies among such women in developing countries have in general not confirmed this fear. And the World Health Organization found that women who were already short of vitamins showed no further decrease in measured levels after one year's use of the pill.

Folic acid and Vitamin B_{12} help to produce normal red blood cells. Anaemia due to the shortage of either of these substances has been described in pill-users, but very rarely and then only in women on poor diets. It might in fact have been a coincidence that they were pill-takers. The more frequent kind of anaemia due to shortage of iron is much *less* common. This is explained in the next chapter, by the fact that pill-users tend to have lighter periods and therefore to lose less iron from the body each month in the menstrual blood.

The lowered levels of most vitamins may even be healthy and appropriate as the body adapts to being on the pill. *There is believed to be no true shortage. So pill-users should not take extra vitamins*, whether by an expensive 'pill protection formula' or from any other source. It is likely to be more not less healthy to rely simply on a normal diet, preferably including plenty of fruit and vegetables.

Taking tablets with extra vitamins might even do harm. For example, it is a quite common practice to take 1 gram a day of Vitamin C, in the (unproven) belief that this will prevent or treat the common cold. *This is not recommended for pill-users*. The reason is that such high doses of Vitamin C *increase* the amount of ethinyloestradiol (page 43) absorbed in the digestive system. This is not good. It has the effect of turning a low-dose pill into a high-dose one, and results in more marked effects on the body chemistry—especially the clotting factors. This breaks that working rule on page 87.

Interestingly, intermittent use of a 1-gram daily dose of Vitamin C has been found to cause breakthrough bleeding each time it is stopped. This is only to be expected, because stopping the Vitamin C is like changing from a higher- to a lower-dose variety of pill, which commonly causes a small amount of bleeding, due to hormone withdrawal (see page 72).

If you are a strong believer in the value of Vitamin C, and insist on taking it, there is one thing you can do: *if you take each drug at a different time, at least four hours apart,* the Vitamin C can no longer increase the absorption of the oestrogen from the gut. If you smoke, new research does show that extra Vitamin C (even then, best taken as citrus fruits or drinks) helps to counteract some bad effects of cigarettes on the arteries.

See pages 108 and 128 for more about *pyridoxine* and *folic acid.*

Retention of fluid and weight gain

This occurs more in some women than others, and is due to some complicated adjustments to body chemistry among pill-users. Except in certain types of heart and kidney disease (in which extra fluid can be dangerous and your doctor would not normally be recommending the pill) this seems to be quite harmless. It does, however, cause some of the weight gain for which the pill is often blamed, perhaps about 1 or 2 kilograms or so, just due to extra water being in the body. This is very temporary and the weight is lost if the pill is stopped. Some users notice that they shed the extra weight regularly during the 7-day break from pill-taking each month. Extra water is also kept in the body, for rather similar reasons, regularly towards the end of the normal menstrual cycle and in early pregnancy.

Weight gain after going on the pill can also result from an actual increase in body fat. This is largely due to an increase in appetite, particularly during the first three months. Watching your intake of calories is the only real answer to this: though easier said than done!

Gaining weight is one of the things which most puts women off the pill. Yet in one study of a modern brand, as many women (15 per cent) actually lost weight as gained it, the remaining 70 per cent staying about the same.

Disorders of the circulatory system: bloodstream, heart, arteries, and veins

Most of this next section has to do with one basic problem known as thrombosis, which is the formation of blood clots in arteries or veins. This causes most of the very rare major troubles blamed on the pill. But thrombosis is also more likely in pregnancy, which is of course avoided by taking the pill.

* *The ability to clot is a most important function of the blood*

Without it even a small injury to a blood-vessel could lead to the injured person bleeding to death. But the oestrogen of the pill tends to cause an increase in the blood levels of most of the important clotting factors and to reduce the amount of an important factor (anti-thrombin III) which tends to stop the clotting process. The pill also changes the functioning of the blood platelets. These are small particles which, among other things, have the ability to stick to each other at the start of clot formation. The tendency to platelet aggregation, as this process is called, is increased in heavy smokers.

* These, among other changes, make clotting more likely to happen where it is *not* wanted, namely in uninjured arteries and veins. Yet if the changes occur to some extent in all pill-users, why do so few ever get any kind of thrombosis? An important reason for this seems to be that other systems are brought into play: particularly the one called fibrinolysis whereby any blood clots which appear in the circulation are removed as fast as they are formed. Thus often along with the increased tendency to clotting because of the raised clotting factors, there is at the same time a sufficient improvement of this process for getting rid of blood clots. Good health demands a balance between the two mechanisms. In pill-users it seems that this balance tends to be achieved by resetting them both at a higher level. Very

interestingly, it has been found that this balancing increase in fibrinolysis tends not to happen in smokers, especially heavy smokers. If such women then take the pill, their increased clotting factors will no longer be counteracted by a better clot-removing system. This, along with the effect of smoking on platelets, may be part of the reason why the most recent research cannot show an effect of the pill to increase the risk of thrombosis of the type occurring in *arteries*, unless the women also smoke (see below).

Clotting can occur either in veins or arteries. Because these are everywhere in the body and the effect of a clot is to block the flow of blood at that point, what exactly happens will depend on whereabouts the blockage has occurred. If an *artery* is involved, then the part of the body supplied by that artery may lose its blood supply altogether and it can be severely damaged. *Veins* take the blood at low pressure back from different parts of the body to the heart. If they are blocked by a blood clot the local effects are usually less severe. The trouble with venous clots, however, is that they themselves may move through the bloodstream, by a process known as *embolism*, and finish up somewhere else, where they can do more harm. This is most commonly somewhere in the lungs.

Clotting in veins (venous thrombosis)

This was the first clotting problem to be linked with the pill and was recognized first in the large veins of the leg: the so-called deep veins. Given an increased level of clotting factors, the reason that clotting tends to occur in the legs is because the rate of flow tends to be slowest there. Lack of flow (stasis) is particularly likely if the pill-user is overweight, takes insufficient exercise, and above all if she is confined to bed by illness, operation, or accident.

As a rule, thrombosis of a deep vein shows up by pain and tenderness in the calf of the affected leg, aggravated if someone bends the ankle joint upwards. There may also be obvious swelling on that side. Whether or not there are these symptoms in the leg, rarely a piece of the blood clot may break off. After travelling in the great veins and right through the heart it can finish up in the lung (*pulmonary embolism*). If the clot is big enough, this can—very rarely—even be fatal by stopping the blood flow through the lungs altogether. Otherwise there is a sharp pain in the chest, usually on one side or the other, worse at every breath, and sometimes a small amount of blood may be coughed up. The treatment, apart from stopping the pill *immediately, and for ever*, is usually by admission to hospital for treatment designed to 'thin' the blood. This is done by drugs called anti-coagulants, and sometimes by other treatments which can dissolve clots. Most exceptionally, in a severe case, an urgent operation on the chest to remove the clot may be required.

Like all the conditions in this chapter and the next, this chain of events can also happen in women who have never taken a pill in their lives, and in men. However, it is roughly *twice* as likely among women taking the pill as among non-users. The risk is connected with the oestrogen content of any pill.

Apart from the pill itself, the factors which seem to make clotting in veins more likely are: obesity; confinement to bed; recent surgical operation (especially bone surgery); pregnancy; increasing age; and past *personal* history, or *family* history, of any form of thrombosis. Diabetes and high blood pressure are other factors. Thrombosis in veins is actually less common in people who have the blood group O. Fortunately, group O is in fact the commonest one, possessed by about half the population. Smoking is not connected with this kind of thrombosis, unlike the type discussed below, in arteries. The increased risk due to the pill is much reduced in modern low-oestrogen varieties: it is not related to duration of use, and it goes away quickly if the pill is stopped—certainly within about 4–6 weeks.

If there is a history in your family of a close relative (parent, brother, or sister) who had a blood clot in the leg or the lung under the age of 40, tell your doctor. Detailed blood clotting studies ought ideally to be arranged: if they are not available or prove to be abnormal you should use another method of family planning, not the pill.

A note on varicose veins

Many women and some doctors wrongly think that you should always avoid the pill if you have varicose veins even if they have never caused any problems. This is just not so: the type of blood clotting I am describing here which can be dangerous starts in the *deep* veins, particularly of the calf.

Many women who would like to use the pill are frightened to take it because of really almost microscopic varicose veins. Some of them actually finish up with the tragedy of an unwanted pregnancy. *Provided* the other risk factors which were listed above do not apply, and especially if you are not overweight, moderate varicose veins with no signs of any past thrombosis need not stop you going on the pill. You may notice that they become a little more prominent and that you perhaps get some aching in your legs, particularly if you have to stand a long time. However, should you, without any obvious explanation for it (such as an injection or pressure from a plaster cast), ever have suffered in any vein of the body from 'phlebitis', which involves thrombosis, you should avoid or stop the pill. As a general rule, you should also *never take it in future in case you were to have a clot somewhere more important next time.*

You should stop the pill four weeks before *varicose vein surgery* (page 174). The same caution is needed for anyone having *injection treatment* for veins, since this works by causing clotting in them, after which the body causes scarring to seal them up. To prevent this being overdone, you should stop the pill a month beforehand, stay off it during the period that you visit your doctor's surgery or the out-patient department for the treatment, and ideally for three months afterwards. During all this time you will of course need to use some other reliable method of family planning. As the clotting was caused deliberately, this treatment should not stop you going on the pill once again, provided your doctor agrees.

Clotting in arteries (arterial thrombosis)

The main reason why clotting in arteries occurs is because of a disease of the walls of the arteries which is often called arteriosclerosis ('hardening of the arteries') or more properly atherosclerosis. This disease affects almost everyone in due course, men usually at a younger age than women. In the more developed countries of the world it has usually started well before the age of 20, and gets more marked as the individual gets older, especially if he or she is a smoker. It affects some much more than others, and one important factor seems to be high levels or an abnormal ratio of the levels of the various blood lipids mentioned earlier.

The changes in blood-clotting factors, especially those which affect the blood platelets, are also important. Given the fact that the walls of an artery have been damaged by atherosclerosis, clotting on the surface of the roughened bit of the wall can then occur and eventually this may block up the artery altogether. If it is an important one, such as an artery supplying the heart, the results can be very serious—i.e. a coronary thrombosis or heart attack. If the artery supplies part of the brain, then a cerebral thrombosis may result with the production of one type of stroke.

Once again it is important to realize that any of these events can happen, unfortunately, to women who have never taken a single pill in their lives and to *men*. In pill-takers recent studies have found the risk to be undetectably small unless they also smoke, or have one of the other recognized 'risk factors' discussed below.

Coronary thrombosis (heart attack)

The pill is only one of many factors which make heart attacks more likely, and indeed a less important one than some of those in the list which follows.

Risk factors for arterial thrombosis:

1. *Abnormal blood fats.* As discussed earlier, there is a group of people who have a 'high blood cholesterol' or other blood fat problem from birth and should never take the pill. Many of them know about this, but a lot more do not: the appropriate blood tests need to be done if a near-relative (especially mother, father, sister, or brother) suffered a first heart attack or other arterial thrombosis under the age of 45. This history means more if the relative was a non-smoker. (See also pages 87, 90, and 155–6.)

2. *Diabetes requiring treatment.*

3. *High blood pressure, bad enough for treatment.* A past history of the blood pressure going up in pregnancy—now called

pregnancy-related hypertension—is also a strong factor. However, the pill does not add any greater *increment* of thrombosis risk than it does to women without the pregnancy history, and the risk of blood pressure going up on the pill is also no higher. So the pill need not be avoided if you have this history. It will just be important to keep a closer eye than usual on your blood pressure, especially in the early months of pill-taking. (See page 179.)

4. *Cigarette-smoking*, especially if heavy. In one study which included 64 women under 40 who suffered heart attacks, 60 were smokers. Only 17 were pill-users, all of them smokers. Thus there were no cases in pill-users unless they also smoked.

5. *Increasing age*, especially beyond 35 in smokers.

6. *Obesity* is also a factor increasing the risk, but it possibly does not act independently. In other words, many experts believe that it tends to go along with or have a hand in causing some of the other factors mentioned such as abnormal blood fats, or diabetes, and these explain the extra risk.

7. Another factor is the possession of a *blood group other than group O*. (The other groups in this system are groups A, B, and AB.) In other words, blood group O seems to give a bit of protection against clotting in arteries as well as veins. Though not routinely tested for, the presence of group O can help tip the balance about using the pill in a borderline case—e.g. a woman with one or more of risk factors 1–6.

The important thing to understand about these factors is that if more than one applies to a particular woman there is a dramatic increase in the risk she runs. Let us take as an example a healthy 25-year-old woman who is not a diabetic, has normal blood fat levels and blood pressure, and does not smoke. If she starts to smoke cigarettes her chances of a coronary are something like 3 times greater than before, depending on how many she smokes. But if she swallows a daily pill and also smokes more than 15 cigarettes a day her risk goes up by at most 2 for the pill *multiplied* by 3 (for the smoking), to 6 times the initial value. Double that if her daily consumption is 30 cigarettes.

What would happen if she had a third risk factor, say a sufficiently raised blood pressure to add a further 5-times risk? Multiplying again, she would then be 5 times 12 or 60 times less safe than a healthy non-smoker with normal blood pressure not taking the pill.

All these figures are very approximate. Research so far cannot give precise estimates of the risks, and they are only averages anyway, whereas every pill-user is a unique individual.

The risk factors in the list above are also relevant (some more than others) to the causation of other forms of thrombosis in arteries—see below. If you look again at the list it will be clear that there is not a lot you can do about several of them. If you have that high blood cholesterol condition which runs in families, or you are unlucky enough to have diabetes, or have now developed high blood pressure—apart from taking your dietary advice and treatment, relaxing a bit, and perhaps taking more exercise, there is not much you can do about the situation. Nor, more's the pity, can you make yourself younger or change your blood group! If you are overweight you ought to be able to return to the ideal weight for your height by dieting, and this is well worth doing anyway. But the number one risk factor that you can in theory do something about, and which is perhaps the most common and may well be one of the most important, is of course *smoking*. As one researcher has said, summarizing a lot of research by experts in many different countries, coronary thrombosis 'in otherwise healthy pre-menopausal women is almost exclusively an illness of cigarette smokers'.

Clotting in the arteries of the brain (cerebral thrombosis)

This can cause one type of *stroke*: very suddenly the person notices weakness leading to loss of all sensation or the ability to move the muscles on one side of the body; or loss of the power of normal speech. Other symptoms may be produced, depending on which part of the brain is damaged. Sometimes there can be almost complete recovery, but some people are left with permanent loss of power or feeling on one side and perhaps impairment of their speech. Stroke in general is very rare among women under the age of 40. However, we now know that the pill increases the risk, both of this type of stroke and of the type due to bleeding into the brain which can often be very difficult to distinguish from it (described below). Interestingly, although the thrombosis occurs in arteries, no connection between this type of stroke and smoking has yet been shown—but see below.

Strokes caused by bleeding

Two varieties of strokes due to bleeding appear to be more likely among pill-users. One is *intracerebral haemorrhage* (bleeding into the substance of the brain) causing damage and similar symptoms to those after thrombosis in the arteries supplying the same part of the brain. The other is known as *subarachnoid haemorrhage*, or bleeding into the cerebro-spinal fluid which surrounds the brain and spinal cord. This type leads to rapid and often prolonged loss of consciousness, from which the patient may or may not make a slow and not always complete recovery following medical or surgical treatment. Both these rare catastrophes are due to a localized weakness of the wall of an artery in the brain giving way. There seems to be a very clear link between these strokes due to bleeding and smoking. In one study, eight of nine current or past users of the pill who had a subarachnoid haemorrhage were also smokers. High blood pressure, whether or not the pill has ever been used, is even more important. Some people are born with a weakness somewhere in a brain artery: raised pressure in that artery will make it more likely to give way. A British study concluded from all the known facts that subarachnoid haemorrhage 'should thus probably not be regarded as a serious cause for concern in healthy women using the pill, provided their blood pressure remains in the normal range' (see pages 102–3).

Prevention of strokes—'beware rising blood pressure and bad or strange migraines' . . .

Sometimes a stroke may be avoidable by prompt action, mainly by stopping the pill if ever the blood pressure is found to be too high (pages 103, 172, 179) and also if certain unusual symptoms appear.

Among *migraine* sufferers, a few notice while taking the pill a marked change in the pattern of their migraine, so that it becomes more *focal* as it is called, with clear-cut localization of their symptoms to one part or function of the body. Along with (or sometimes without) the migraine headache itself, characteristic symptoms have occurred in some women, some hours or a few days before an actual stroke occurred. They include:

sudden onset of short-lived but marked tingling, loss of sensation or weakness affecting one side of the body or one limb only;

complete loss briefly of one half of the field of vision;

a fleeting difficulty in speaking normally;

a first-ever shaking attack like an epileptic fit; or,

loss of consciousness.

NB *Headache on one side of the head is not on the list, as this is normal in migraine; and neither flashing lights nor general blurring of vision means focal migraine.*

Focal symptoms just might mean that there is a temporary loss of blood supply to part of the brain. With or without a headache they should be treated as an early warning and the pill stopped at once, probably for ever. It is the oestrogen that matters, since stopping its effects on blood clotting may help prevent blockage to a brain artery from becoming permanent. This means the woman can switch right away to either the progestogen-only pill or an injectable like DMPA (see Chapter 8). See pages 111–12 for more about migraine.

However, strokes are very uncommon, so there could well be a quite different explanation in your case. When in doubt, discuss any strange symptoms promptly with your doctor (see page 75).

Thrombosis in other parts of the body

As there are arteries and veins everywhere, so thrombosis can affect other organs than those mentioned so far.

Mesenteric thrombosis is the name given to clotting in an artery or vein which supplies the bowel.

- If a large *artery* is affected an emergency operation may be required to remove dead bowel and stitch together the live parts each side of it.
- If one of the main *veins* leading from the bowel is affected, the results can vary between nothing, because the other veins take over, and serious, because of interference with the flow of blood taking absorbed food substances to the

liver. There have also been isolated reports of blockage in the veins the other side of the liver, on the way back to the heart.

The eyes. Rarely, venous or arterial thrombosis (*or* bleeding) can cause damage to a part or all of the retina (the light-sensitive part at the back of the eye). This causes loss of vision in the affected eye, which is a disaster if it should be permanent: but it may be only temporary if the pill is stopped and expert treatment started at once.

Raised blood pressure

In most pill-users there is a measurable slight rise in blood pressure. However, in only about one woman out of every 50 who take the pill does this reach the level at which doctors term it hypertension. The reason why the rest are not more affected is still not clear. There are certainly changes in the circulation and in body chemistry (see Table 4) which may be involved, but those which have been measured often happen also in pill-users without a particularly high blood pressure. Some individuals are known to be more prone generally to raised blood pressure: those with a history of it in their family, those who have had kidney disease, and some black people. The pill may 'bring out' the blood pressure problem in such women, particularly as they get older. One group of researchers has also shown that women with hypertension on the pill have higher levels of the hormone ethinyloestradiol in their blood than other pill-users. So perhaps the few individuals who develop this problem are exceptional in the way their bodies absorb and handle the pill's hormones.

Whatever the reason, there are two main points about raised blood pressure. First, it usually does *not* make you feel at all unwell. Second, when large groups of both men and women with even very mild hypertension have been followed up, they have not remained as healthy over the years as comparison groups with entirely normal blood pressure readings. Blood pressure seems to be linked with nearly all the diseases of the circulatory system and is often a feature of people who later suffer thrombosis in veins, heart attacks, and strokes. It also has the risk itself of becoming uncontrollable, even with drugs, leading to malignant hypertension which is very rare but fatal.

As raised blood pressure is something that can be readily detected, it can be used as an early warning sign of other circulation problems with which it seems to be linked. It is obviously vital, therefore, if you use the pill that you have your blood pressure taken regularly. The pressure is measured in the main artery of the arm, the brachial artery. The highest (systolic) pressure reached in that artery during each pumping action of the heart is the first figure that doctors quote, and should not normally be above 140 mm of mercury. The lowest pressure reached before the next heartbeat is the other measurement, the diastolic pressure, and should not be above 90 mm. Several readings above these levels are necessary before mild hypertension is diagnosed. Careful medical supervision is then required, and if there are any other risk factors the pill should be discontinued. The pill usually has to be stopped anyway if the upper figure reaches 160 mm or the lower 95 mm or more (these figures are those used by the World Health Organization to define clinical hypertension). Just stopping the pill generally brings the blood pressure back to normal within a month or two. Further treatment (with drugs) is rarely required for women during the child-bearing years. All brands of the *combined* pill tend to cause a recurrence of the problem, and so should be avoided: but the progestogen-only pill and DMPA (page 255) may be tried, often successfully.

The Study of the British Royal College of General Practitioners

Much of the information for this chapter and the next comes from the Oral Contraception Study organized by the Royal College of General Practitioners (RCGP). The Study began in 1968 when about 23,000 pill-users from the practices of 1,400 family doctors all over Britain were matched up with another 23,000 similar women who were not taking the pill. Ever since that time every episode of disease, treated at home or requiring hospital admission, and all pregnancies and of course deaths were recorded. Many women discontinued the pill for one reason or another, so that eventually there were three groups: pill-takers, ex-takers, and never-users. The ex-takers have been studied carefully for any possible harmful effects and also benefits of the pill which might carry on even after it was stopped.

Two similar studies also began in 1968. One, referred to as the Oxford/FPA Study, was organized by the British Family Planning Association working with Professor Vessey of Oxford University. Full details were obtained of all the hospital attendances of 17,032 women who were recruited between 1968 and 1974 from FPA clinics throughout Britain. A little over half the women were on the pill when first seen, the others used the cap or an intra-uterine device (IUD).

The Walnut Creek Study is named after a suburban township near San Francisco, California. Between 1968 and 1972, 16,638 women had a general health check-up provided by the Kaiser-Permanente Medical Care Program at Walnut Creek. They were subsequently followed up until 1977 and their health details were analysed. Those who had used or were currently using the pill were compared with the remainder, whose methods of contraception (if any) were not recorded. (This is a weakness of the Walnut Creek Study and applies to the RCGP one as well.)

The findings of these three groups of researchers differ in some details but agree in most important respects. As the RCGP group studied the largest number, its results more commonly have statistical significance. But most weight is given in this book, as it should be, to those findings which are *confirmed*

(a) by other studies (such as the other two mentioned); and

(b) by other types of research, in different populations.

The RCGP researchers concluded that the overall death rate due to diseases of the circulation was greater in 'ever-users' (55) of the pill than 'never-users' (10). The numbers in brackets are the actual numbers of deaths, totalling 65. That is not a large number out of the 46,377 studied, for an average of just under seven years (322,438 woman-years of observation).

Among current users the RCGP researchers could find no firm evidence of an effect of duration of use on the risk of circulatory disease. This is a good piece of news which emerged only in their 1981 report, and later evidence remains broadly reassuring.

The overall death rates hide within them very different risks for different sub-groups of pill-users (see page 164). As the main serious problem is arterial disease, the women chiefly at risk are those with any of the risk factors listed on pages 97–8.

Smoking, age, and the pill—THE PILL MAKES YOUR SMOKING EVEN MORE DANGEROUS

All studies agree that the pill's hazards are heavily concentrated in cigarette smokers and older women. Smoking has been proved to do two things: not only does it increase the risk of getting an arterial disease, it also makes the attack more likely to be fatal.

The Walnut Creek researchers were even more emphatic. They could show the risk for pill-users who were also smokers, and for non-pill-users who smoked. In the absence of smoking, however, they could demonstrate no effect of the pill at all on circulatory disease risk. The more recent (1989) reports about heart attacks by the RCGP and the Oxford/FPA Studies say exactly the same thing. Of course this does not prove complete safety for non-smoking pill-takers: but if the risk is now undetectable it must have become mighty small. Why? Partly it seems because prescribers now know better who should avoid the pill and partly because we have available much safer brands than before.

26 October 1989 was a red-letter day for pill-users! On that day the facts in the last paragraph, plus a greater understanding of the BENEFITS of the pill for older women led the relevant Medical Advisory Committee of the American Food and Drugs Administration (FDA) to make an extremely important statement. They advised that *for women free of all risk factors including smoking there need no longer be any upper age limit for the pill.* This instantly helped a large group of women who had previously been told they must use another method from age 35 or perhaps 40 up to the menopause. (See pages 189–92, 222, 258 for more on this, including the best pill for such women.)

But there was of course *no change in the upper age limit for smokers: still 35 years.*

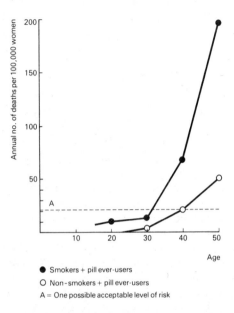

Fig. 13 Influence of pill-use, smoking, and age on overall death rates due to diseases of the circulation. Based on figures from the RCGP report (1981)

Why 'of course'? Take a look at Figure 13. Notice how heavy smoking effectively makes you up to 10 years older than you really are. Whatever level of risk a pill-user is prepared to accept, if she is a smoker she will reach it sooner. In the example shown, an overall annual risk of 20 per 100,000 women (i.e. betting odds on survival 5,000 to 1) is reached at about age 32, rather than 39 for a non-smoker.

The Figure is based mainly on old-style 50 mcg pills, so there is every reason to believe the difference would be even greater using modern pills and so would strongly support the FDA statement just quoted.

To avoid the pill and continue puffing away, in response to the facts about the relative dangers of the pill and of smoking, is to 'strain out a mosquito and swallow a camel'; or a bit like a stunt motor-cyclist refusing to play golf for fear of injury.

Smoking in effect ages your arteries and increases the risk of most diseases of the circulation for all women (and men), regardless of their method of family planning. On top of that smokers are accepting some pretty frightening hazards, including bronchitis, gangrene of the legs, and cancer of the lung, larynx, bladder, and cervix. (The last two, and others not listed, are by the effect of chemicals absorbed from the smoke into the bloodstream, see page 50.) One in four smokers die earlier than they otherwise would of a disease related to smoking: like Russian roulette with four rather than six chambers in the revolver!

Of course, you can get injured by a golf ball, and the pill certainly does have problems. But if you put together all the problems mentioned in this chapter and the next, it still does not put the pill into the same league as the cigarette. And if you add the pill to your cigarettes, you make smoking even more dangerous than it would otherwise be.

The obvious if difficult answer is to get rid of the smoking. *It is always worth giving up*. The potentially dangerous changes in the blood of smokers, two of which were mentioned on page 78, revert to normal quite rapidly. After a few years ex-smokers have no greater chance of dying than lifetime non-smokers.

By stopping smoking they even benefit those around them. Breathing other people's cigarette smoke is dangerous for non-smokers, especially young children (not to mention the risks to unborn babies if their mothers smoke).

Oddly enough most surveys show that pill-users are *more* likely than average to be smokers! *Yet ideally no pill-user, whether aged 20 or 35, should ever smoke cigarettes*. Non-users of the pill would benefit as well, of course. Indeed, if this book were to persuade just a dozen women to give up cigarettes and, better still, a few more to help their husbands to give up and, best of all, others to persuade their children not to take up the habit in the first place, it would have achieved something!

5

....

Other effects of the pill

This chapter is like a conducted tour of the systems of the body, starting at the head and more or less working downwards. At the end there are some miscellaneous subjects which do not readily fit in elsewhere. Conditions which were dealt with in the last chapter because they were primarily caused by a disorder of the circulation are only cross-referenced. This applies, for example, to strokes, which are disorders of the brain and central nervous system but are caused by arterial disease and have therefore already been discussed.

Within each system, the more common known unwanted effects are considered before those that are rare, followed by the good known effects. And as before *asterisks* (*) mean more detail than you may want.

The brain and central nervous system

Depression (see also page 182)

This is a most complicated subject. Firstly, depression which comes on regularly pre-menstrually in the normal menstrual cycle is, naturally, most commonly improved by the pill. Secondly, in the Oxford/FPA study (page 103) there was shown to be no increase in the risk of severe depression; or indeed of any mental disorder so bad as to require a specialist opinion or admission to hospital. However, most researchers do find that a few more than the expected number of women using the pill complain of mild or moderate depression. And there could sometimes be an explanation in body chemistry because, as shown in Table 4 (page 88), pyridoxine (Vitamin B_6) levels are lowered in the blood of some depressed pill-users. This vitamin is known to be involved in producing certain amines of the brain, substances which affect how it functions. Depressed pill-users with lowered levels of pyridoxine, but not those who were equally depressed with normal blood levels of the vitamin, did notice an improvement in one study in which thay were given extra amounts of this vitamin every day. But the experts are very divided as to whether it is a good idea to make it a routine that pill-users who complain of depression are given pyridoxine. The treatment would not benefit those who did not lack this vitamin. Those who lack it might be helped, and some doctors therefore prescribe it. A dose of 50 mg per day is plenty and should do no harm so far as we know. Foods that are rich in pyridoxine include wheatgerm, liver, meats, fish, milk, bananas, and peanuts.

As a matter of fact, there are reasons for questioning how much of the increase in depression reported among pill-users is really due to the pill. The excess rate in the RCGP Study was only about 30 per cent. Now depression is very common, and affects practically everyone—men as well as women—at some time or another. The pill is commonly used, so depression and use of the pill might well come together by coincidence. The pill may be blamed when really the depression is due to a combination of factors in the woman's whole life. But these may be so hard to tackle that it is very understandable to hope that stopping the pill will be the answer.

Another point is that the pill users in the RCGP study had to go to their doctor more often than the non-users just to pick up their prescriptions, and so would be more likely to mention the fact if they were depressed. This could lead to a bias against the pill. If for the sake of argument we blame the pill for the whole 30 per cent excess noted among users, that still means that out of every 130 depressed pill-users 100 cannot really blame their depression on the method.

The pill has such a reputation for causing depression that this is one of the commonest reasons given by women who stop using it. Many could be giving it up unnecessarily. (Some of them may end up with a very depressing unplanned pregnancy.) Having said that, it is still true that there is a group of women who do find that their mood improves dramatically when they stop taking the pill and worsens whenever they start it again.

So, what should you do if you become depressed while taking the pill? The best advice is to discuss the whole matter with your doctor. Moving to an ultra-low-dose pill may help, or to one with one of the new progestogens (see page 155), and this is certainly worth a try if this is the only problem, before transferring to another method altogether. Your doctor might suggest treatment with pyridoxine, or perhaps with some anti-depressant or tranquillizer: if so, be sure to discuss whether the pill and the new medicine might interfere with each other's actions (see page 67). Finally, take heart from the fact that mild and moderate attacks of depression are not 'life sentences' and usually you can expect to feel better before too many months have gone by.

Loss of libido (interest in sex)

This can happen because of depression, but also for other reasons. Few people realize how common it is, especially after a recent pregnancy. Many women start taking the pill after having a baby, and blame the pill for the depression and loss of libido that follows when it is really part of the post-natal 'blues'. Another possible explanation is that some women still feel that sex is primarily for babies, and as taking the pill makes pregnancy extremely unlikely, they lose their interest in love-making. However, these two explanations are not the whole story. Like depression, it is undeniable that some cases are indeed caused by the pill. One simple diagnosis can be that the vagina seems drier in some women due to some loss of the natural lubrication. If this is a problem it can be helped considerably by using something like a jelly lubricant regularly before intercourse. Actually, many women report an improvement in their sex lives once they go on the pill and most surveys have shown that, in general, pill-users have more intercourse each month. This may be because the pill avoids the 'turn-off' effect which some couples find with alternative methods. Or it may reduce the regular loss of libido due to pre-menstrual tension which many women get in their (so-called) normal menstrual cycles.

So once again, take heart if you do go through a phase of lost interest in sex on the pill. Discuss the whole matter with your doctor. Transferring to a more oestrogen-dominant pill (page 204) or one containing a new-type progestogen may help. In a few cases the doctor may recommend some special sessions of counselling for you and your partner, to improve your general and sexual relationship. Only rarely should it be necessary for you to give up the pill solely for this reason.

Migraine

Migraines are periodic, very variable, often severe, and usually one-sided headaches, linked with sickness or actual vomiting. There are commonly other symptoms like intolerance of bright lights or noise and short-lived disturbances of vision. There is much disagreement between doctors as to what causes migraines. In many women they are thought to be due to an alteration in the responsiveness of the blood-vessels of the brain to those special substances called amines (see page 108). The pill like the natural hormones of the menstrual cycle may cause migraines by affecting these amines, perhaps partly because of its effects on the vitamin pyridoxine. Another important factor can be amines coming in the diet: for instance, cheese, chocolate, sherry, and red wine are all rich in one of them (tyramine), and can all precipitate migraine in some women. Allergy may also be a factor in some people; smoking is an important factor; and three out of every four migraine sufferers have a family history of some relative with the same problem.

A very few women on the pill actually report some improvement in their migraines. Rather more say that the pill makes their attacks more frequent, or has even brought this problem on for the very first time. One of the most common patterns is for the headaches to occur during the seven days while the woman is not taking tablets, probably because of the sudden drop in the hormone levels. A possible short-term solution, provided there are no 'focal' symptoms (see page 101), is then to take an ultra-low-dose combined pill on the tricycle basis described on page 52. For this purpose, a pill from near the bottom of one of the 'ladders' in Chapter 7 (Figure 17, pages 190–1) should be chosen. Transferring to a progestogen-only pill (Chapter 8) can sometimes help as this is also taken every day with no pill-free weeks.

For all types of migraine, avoiding various foods, cigarettes and stressful situations can help. It can be a miserable complaint. In practice, the majority of sufferers from true migraines give the pill up altogether. This is indeed usually recommended for those who develop migraines for the first time while taking the pill, or who require to take ergotamine-containing drugs during attacks. The pill should also be stopped immediately and you should discuss the matter promptly with a doctor if:

(a) any migraine worsens to produce a headache which simply gets worse and worse and worse as the hours go by (crescendo migraine) or

(b) you begin to get very *localized* or so-called 'focal' symptoms (but *not* just a one-sided headache).

Examples of the kind of symptoms and the reasons for acting promptly in this way are given on page 101.

Headaches

Ordinary (non-migraine) headaches are extremely common in women not taking the pill and also in men. Thus it is hard to know how much the pill can really be blamed for the headaches pill-users may get. After depression, this was the second commonest reason women gave for giving up the method in the RCGP Study. Apart from taking pain-killers if necessary, the treatment is to use the very lowest-dose pill that suits you in other ways. If they happen mostly during the pill-free week, your doctor may again recommend the tricycle regime (page 52). You could change the progestogen (transferring to a different 'ladder'—see Figure 17, pages 190–1); or possibly transfer to the progestogen-only pill. It would be rather unusual for you to have to give up the method for this reason alone.

*Epilepsy

There is no suggestion that the pill *causes* epilepsy. In fact many sufferers report fewer attacks when they go on the pill. However, a very few do get more frequent epileptic attacks, and may have to give up the method. There is also the distinct possibility that the tablets they take to control fits may interfere with the hormones of the pill once absorbed into the body, and reduce the protection it provides against pregnancy (see page 67). There are a couple of anti-epileptic drugs (sodium valproate and clonazepam) which do not do this, but they are not ideal for all patients.

Those who are on the other treatments, the liver-enzyme inducers shown in Table 3, page 70, should discuss the whole matter with their doctor. They may decide to use another method such as the IUD, but the pill can still be some women's best choice of family planning method. If so it should definitely be one of the ones containing 50 mcg of oestrogen from Table 10 (page 188). Since the pill-free interval is the contraceptively risky time (page 62), I recommend that long-term users of medicines which weaken the pill simply have fewer of them. In other words the woman *tricycles the pill* (page 52), taking three or even four packs of pills in a row, *without any breaks* at all. After that a shortened gap between runs of packets is logical, usually 5 days. The woman should be more than usually careful to take her tablets regularly and will also have to report promptly back to the surgery or clinic should she develop 'breakthrough' bleeding on tablet-taking days.

* If so, occasionally she might even be prescribed two pills a day. This to her body would only be the same as taking one pill, of course. It is a bit like 'climbing up a down escalator'. The extra hormones are being got rid of faster by the speeding up of the liver's metabolism (because of the anti-epileptic drug). This leaves only the same amount in the system as other pill-takers would get from one pill a day.

See also pages 99–100 for *strokes*.

*Chorea

This rare condition causes the patient to make strange uncontrolled fidgety movements of the head, arms, and legs. It may have occurred in the past, during an attack of rheumatic fever or in pregnancy. With or without such a history, it has been found to happen in one or two pill-users. It always clears up if the pill is discontinued.

In the 1970s neurologists reported that pill-use was more likely among those very few young thin women who gave a strange story. They noticed headache and a blind spot in their field of vision on exercise. If they also had a swelling of the optic nerves when the light-sensitive retina at the back of their eyes was examined (papilloedema), the condition was diagnosed as BICP. It usually got better if the pill was stopped, following rule 8 on page 75. The problem seems no longer to be reported with modern ultra-low-dose brands.

The Eyes

Problems with contact lenses

Some contact-lens-users find that their eyes get sore for the first time when they start the pill. A possible reason seems to be that there is a slight increase in the amount of fluid in the cornea (the transparent covering in front of the iris). If the eyes do become really uncomfortable, it is important that vanity does not make you persevere too long and you take the lenses out to give the eyes a rest. (It is possible otherwise to damage the surface of the sensitive cornea.) Then you should discuss the matter with your optician. Although this complaint is definitely less common with modern lenses, and with modern ultra-low-dose pills, a few women do have to make a straight choice: either the pill or their contact lenses.

*Other eye problems

A couple of reports suggest that long-term pill-users cannot see the colour blue as well as some non-users. This was something that showed up on specialized testing, and not something of which the women themselves complained.

Quite a range of other eye problems have been reported in women who were taking the pill. In many of them pill-use may well have been coincidental. For example, no link has been proved between the pill and glaucoma (in which there is a rise in the pressure of the fluid within the eyeball).

See also page 101 for *retinal thrombosis/bleeding*.

The respiratory system: air passages and lungs

Allergic rhinitis (hay fever)

This can sometimes become a problem for the first time when a woman starts taking the pill. The pill seems to be able to alter the immune systems of the body (see Table 4 and page 137), so this could be a genuine effect of the pill, though not yet proved to be so.

Asthma

This does not appear to start for the first time more commonly in pill-users than other women, probably because it is a problem which tends to run in families and rarely starts for the first time in adults. Some women with asthma notice that their symptoms are improved on the pill, some that they are worsened. In the majority there is no change. So if the method suits in other ways it is well worth a try.

See also page 94 for *pulmonary embolism*.

Disorders of the digestive system

Nausea (queasiness)

With modern pills this is quite uncommon except in women who are underweight—including therefore many pill-users from the developing world. If it occurs, it is experienced particularly during the first few days of pill-taking, from each of the first two or three packets, and then may disappear for ever. Perseverance, or taking the pills with a drink and a little food at bedtime so that you are asleep when the symptom appears, should be all you have to do. Otherwise see your doctor or clinic for a lower dose of *oestrogen* in the pill.

Do not forget the possibility that the nausea might be due to pregnancy, of course, particularly if it appears for the first time after several months' use of the method. Arrange a test if in any doubt.

Duodenal ulcers

Here we have a possible good effect of the pill. Both the RCGP

Study and the Oxford/FPA Study are agreed that women on the pill were less likely than non-users to require treatment for severe indigestion due to this type of ulcer. However, it is hard to rule out the possibility that the anxious person who is prone to get such ulcers will also be particularly unlikely to use the pill.

*Crohn's disease

This uncommon bowel disease causes pain and diarrhoea. It appears that one form of it (non-granulomatous Crohn's) occurs more frequently in pill-takers; if the pill is stopped, complete recovery is the rule. The pill can however (continue to) be used whenever it is not thought to be connected with the trouble, obviously with careful supervision. Despite the diarrhoea the hormones seem to be absorbed normally. So there is no need to take a stronger brand.

See page 101 for *mesenteric thrombosis*.

The liver and gall-bladder

The liver has many special *receptors* for sex hormones, and therefore its many functions are often influenced by the pill (see Table 4). The alterations, in clotting factors and blood fats for example, mean that the liver is probably at the back of most of the unwanted effects of the pill which occur elsewhere. Many side-effects might become even more rare if the pill was not a pill at all! i.e. if it was taken instead by one of the new non-oral routes—see pages 224–5, 230–3.

Fortunately in most women the liver itself is not apparently harmed in any way. Exceptions are below, and on page 145: *liver tumours*.

Jaundice

This is the liver disease which makes the skin and the eyeballs go a yellow colour. The reason for this is an increase in the amount of a yellow substance called bilirubin in the blood. Bilirubin is normally present in the bile, which is a fluid produced by the liver and carried in ducts to the small bowel. This fluid helps in the digestion of food. A very small number of pill-users may get jaundice of a special type, due to blockage within the substance of the liver to this flow of bile. There is then back-pressure so some of the bile spills over into the general bloodstream, causing yellowness and also itching. The same type of jaundice can occur sometimes in late pregnancy. In fact, if you had this jaundice in pregnancy, or if you had troublesome itching in late pregnancy which often has the same explanation, then you will be advised to avoid using the combined pill altogether in case it causes a recurrence.

Gallstones

The gall-bladder is the reservoir for bile. Bile is a very saturated solution, and it has been shown that the hormones of the pill tend to make it even more saturated. In a few women this can lead to crystals separating out, followed by stone formation. The symptoms which may be caused by stones are a type of indigestion or heavy feeling in the upper part of the abdomen, particularly after meals containing a lot of fat. There may also be nausea and actual vomiting. More severe pain or jaundice may lead to hospital admission.

Apart obviously from stopping the pill, treatment can be medical or surgical. Dissolving the stones with special drugs may be successful, otherwise they are removed along with the gall-bladder. Complete recovery of full health is the rule. And after definitive surgery you may well be allowed back on the pill.

The most recent research indicates that it is only during the earliest years of pill-use that there is an increased risk of gallstones. This suggests that the pill only 'brings out' an inborn tendency.

The urinary system

Cystitis and other urinary infections

Cystitis is the name for infection of the bladder. If the urine is cultured in the laboratory, a germ may be grown and the correct treatment then is an antibiotic. An increased tendency to cystitis was found among pill-users in the RCGP Study, but the Oxford/FPA Study did not find this link. This may be because the latter study looked only at infections bad enough to require referral to hospital. Even when there are no symptoms, bacteria are grown more commonly from the urine of pill-users than other women, and this would make actual infections more likely.

Women on the pill tend to have intercourse frequently, and frequent or vigorous love-making can cause cystitis—you may have heard of 'honeymoon cystitis'. Whether or not the pill is truly to blame for such infections, for some women they can be a real problem. If this is so for you, discuss the matter with your doctor. It will probably help to empty your bladder both before and after intercourse and to use a jelly lubricant (see below). You should take plenty of fluids—e.g. 3 litres in 3 hours—when you get an attack. Your doctor may sometimes advise taking a couple of antibiotic tablets shortly before intercourse as a regular preventive routine. Tests for vaginal infections such as thrush (page 119) may also be necessary, as these infections can cause similar symptoms. For more information see the book by Angela Kilmartin (Further reading, page 292) or ask for the Health Education Council leaflet about cystitis.

The reproductive system: (a) Gynaecology

Vaginal discharge

A few women on the pill complain of excessive dryness of the vagina. This can be quite a problem for some, and may be partly responsible for a loss of interest in sex. It can be due to thrush (see below). Or it can mean that a pill with relatively too high a dose of progestogen is being used (see page 204). So you could ask for a change of pill. It may also help to 'slow down' and have a bit more foreplay before intercourse; or occasionally to use a jelly lubricant. Be straight with yourself, though, and with your partner. Could the problem really be more to do with some aspect of your sexual relationship rather than the pill? Maybe some sex counselling would be more important than a change of pill brand.

However, other pill-users complain of an increase in their vaginal discharge. There are several possible causes for this:

1. *Cervical erosion (new name 'cervical ectopy').* 'Erosion' is a most misleading and unfortunate name for a common, quite harmless condition of the cervix. The normal covering of the outer surface of the cervix is what is known as squamous epithelium, i.e. a covering of flattened cells a little like normal skin. The normal lining of the canal that leads up into the main part of the uterus itself is columnar epithelium (upright, box-shaped cells with a lot of mucus-producing glands). All that happens if there is an erosion is that the normal glands lining the canal spread out over the outer part of the cervix. So it is not an 'ulcer', and nothing has been eroded or eaten away! It just looked like that to the doctors who gave it that name, before anyone had looked at its structure under the microscope.

Ectopy (a much better name) is commoner in pill-users than in non-users. The effect of having more of the type of surface which normally only lines the cervical canal is to have more mucus-producing glands: and hence an increase in the normal wetness of the vagina. Many women, pill-users or not, have this without noticing anything, but a few may call it a discharge.

All that is usually necessary is for the doctor to examine you and to take a cervical smear if you are due to have one. If, however, you are finding the amount of discharge a nuisance, perhaps requiring you to use a tampon or pad to control it, then there are very simple and painless out-patient treatments which can be arranged.

2. *Thrush—otherwise known as candida or monilial infection.* All three of these words apply to the same thing. It is due to a little yeast which is a very common inhabitant of the vagina, often in fact living there without causing any symptoms at all. However, it can cause an attack of intense itching of the vagina and vulva and sometimes burning on passing water, with or *without* a curdy, white vaginal discharge. It is more common in pregnancy; after a course of antibiotics; in women with even very mild diabetes; and seemingly in users of the older, high-oestrogen pills. Surprisingly to many, research on more modern pills was summed up in the title of a paper in the *British Journal of Obstetrics and Gynaecology*: '*The pill does not cause thrush.*'

Anyway, if you get this trouble on the pill or off it, it is usually treated with pessaries which are put into the vagina and cream to be applied outside, around the vulva and anus. The treatments are fortunately now available on 'over the counter' sale. If pessaries are not available here is a useful tip: apply the cream to a tampon (any time of the month) to get it high inside. This can be particularly helpful during a period, to prevent recurrences which are often brought on by menstrual bleeding.

In some women thrush is very troublesome, and keeps recurring. They, and also their partners, may then require extra help, perhaps from a clinic for STDs (see pages 23–6).

Trichomonas vaginitis—known as TV

There is some evidence from two British studies that this common STD (page 23), causing an itchy, fluid vaginal discharge, is less frequent than usual among pill-users. However, there is no proof as yet of this beneficial effect.

Pelvic infection

This also is usually due to STD and can seriously damage the uterine tubes, leading to infertility. Researchers in the USA and elswhere have found that pill-users have half the rate of this kind of infection, compared with those using no contraception. This good effect is probably due mainly to the same mucus changes in the cervix which were described on page 46, caused by progestogen. The altered mucus seems to obstruct bacteria as well as sperm (very probably they 'hitch-hike' because they are actually attached to the sperm!). This reduces but does not of course remove the risk of infections like gonorrhoea and chlamydia spreading up to the tubes. But it is not something to rely on—there are better ways of avoiding these sexually transmitted infections (page 23).

* Toxic-shock syndrome

This is caused by a toxin (poison) getting into the bloodstream and is produced by a bacterium, the Staphylococcus, multiplying in the vagina. The condition was given much publicity in the US because of its link with menstrual tampons. It is extremely rare, the more so if women change their tampons frequently. But it is dangerous, and evidence is emerging that pill-users are *less* likely to get it than others.

Ectopic pregnancy

This is the name for a pregnancy in the wrong place—i.e. not in the cavity of the uterus. Described on page 218, it can lead to dangerous internal bleeding. While a woman takes the pill she is (almost) completely protected from this because she is not releasing eggs. Damaged tubes are the main cause of the problem, so she could still get an ectopic later, after stopping the pill. But there again the pill is somewhat protective because, as we have just seen, it reduces the risk of pelvic infection, and worldwide that is the main cause of tubal damage.

* Fibroids

Here we find another *benefit* of the pill. Fibroids are lumps which can grow on the uterus. They are so common that most women get them eventually, though the size can vary from a large pinhead to as big as a football. They consist of muscle and fibrous tissue. You will probably have heard of them as an occasional cause of excessively heavy periods (menorrhagia) in some women in their late thirties or forties, who therefore require a hysterectomy (removal of the uterus). They are not cancerous. Indeed in most women no treatment at all is ever required.

How does the pill affect fibroids? First, there is nothing to suggest the pill causes fibroids to appear in the first place. But in the days of the old-fashioned high-oestrogen brands, in some individuals the fibroids were noticed to grow very rapidly if they started on the pill. The same sudden increase in size is sometimes seen in pregnancy, and both in pregnancy and on the pill a fibroid can suffer what is known as 'red degeneration'. This is due to breakdown of tissue within it and causes pain.

However, the two main prospective studies (the RCGP Study and the Oxford/FPA Study) are now agreed that fibroids are *less* commonly diagnosed in users of low-oestrogen pills than in non-users, and *less* likely if present to require hospital referral.

The heavy periods which lead to the diagnosis of fibroids if they are present simply do not happen on the pill: because the pill almost always diminishes bleeding from the uterus.

If fibroids are diagnosed, one of the more progestogen-dominant brands is best (page 203). In most women the pill reduces the bleeding trouble that they may cause. But because in a few individuals the fibroids may enlarge, women found to have them should have regular examinations whether or not they stay on the pill. These should all preferably be by the same doctor who can notice any change in size. If available, ultrasound scan tests can also help.

*Endometriosis

This is an uncommon condition which is not entirely understood but causes misery to some women. Each month they suffer from a severe aching or bruising pain before and during the period, worsened by intercourse. This is described as being different in type from menstrual cramps, though it can be just as severe. They may also have to be seen by a gynaecologist for medical or perhaps surgical treatment before they can have a baby.

It is due to some of the same kind of tissue which normally lines the uterus being present in the wrong place: such as in the ovaries (where it is one cause of cysts) or elsewhere in the reproductive system, or even further afield. How this endometrium reached these sites is often unexplained. But just as it bleeds in its correct place, in the uterus, so this wrongly situated endometrium bleeds regularly at period times; and bleeding into the tissues causes bruising pain. As in the uterus, the bleeding results from the fall in blood levels of oestrogen and progestogen.

Continuous treatment or tricycling with a high-progestogen combined pill, or with similar hormones, to abolish egg-release and therefore periods, is logical and does help if there already is endometriosis. Recently a few studies have suggested that this condition is also less likely to be diagnosed in the first place among women who take the pill in the ordinary way. Whether this is a genuine bonus effect of the pill has not yet been finally established.

The ovary—cysts on the ovary

Here we have another advantage of the pill: there are certain ovarian cysts (known as functional cysts) which are commoner in women who are not on the combined pill. These are not tumours: they are balloons containing fluid entirely surrounded by a tissue wall, developing within the ovary. They are thought to arise because of minor imbalances of the natural hormones of the menstrual cycle. Most of them start life as a follicle, stimulated to grow by FSH during the first half of the cycle as described in Chapter 2. However, instead of rupturing to release an egg, or simply losing its fluid and virtually disappearing as the other 19 or so stimulated follicles do, the mechanism can go a bit wrong. Instead, a particular follicle can go on accumulating fluid to produce a cyst. This can be quite a big fluid-filled balloon, up to as much as 10 cm or more in size. (The egg it originally contained dies, of course, and is disposed of by the body in the normal way.)

If the same thing happens over several months, several of these cysts can be produced, perhaps on each ovary. Whether single or multiple, such cysts can sometimes cause quite bad pain, including pain on intercourse. They may cure themselves (by rupturing), or rarely lead to an emergency operation—especially if the cyst causes the whole ovary on either side to twist (torsion).

On the pill, however, the ovaries are usually inactive and no follicles are stimulated to accumulate fluid ready for ovulation. Hence things are less likely to go wrong so as to produce this type of cyst. Here is a way that the combined pill may reduce the need for surgery.

There is a suspicion that the very lowest-dose pills may not suppress the activity of follicles so well and so may produce less of this benefit. And the pill described in Chapter 8 actually increases the risk of functional cysts (page 218).

See also page 144 for another enormously important good effect of the pill, on cancer of the ovary.

Effects on the cycle

For most women, almost everything about periods and the

so-called 'normal' cycle is improved. I say so-called 'normal' because so many women suffer some pretty annoying symptoms from their normal cycles. These can be any or all of the following: short cycles (every 3 weeks or so); irregularity; ovulation pain (Mittelschmerz); pre-menstrual tension; painful periods (dysmenorrhoea); heavy periods leading sometimes to anaemia. The 'normal' can be anything but 'nice'. If men suffered similarly, how many would agree to such a catalogue of troubles being called normal, I wonder! However, *since the pill abolishes the natural menstrual cycle altogether* (see Chapter 2), and replaces it with an apparent cycle caused simply by the fact that the pill's hormones are withdrawn for 7 days in each 28, *most of these symptoms are dramatically improved*. So much so that many women can be very reluctant to give up the pill even if they should, perhaps, for reasons like smoking.

1. *Periods*. If you take the pill in the ordinary way, with regular breaks from pill-taking, you will notice that your 'periods' are very *regular* and can be accurately predicted and are usually also much *lighter*. As an extra bonus you are much *less likely to become anaemic*. This is because heavy periods can cause anaemia due to more iron (in the blood) being lost from the body than you are able to take in your diet.

If you normally suffer with *painful periods*, then the chances are also very good that these will be improved if you go on the pill. Indeed, many teenagers are put on it for this reason alone, even when they need no contraception. Period pains are caused by excessive contractions of the uterus, due mainly to substances called prostaglandins, released during the period. It seems that the thinner type of endometrium which develops in women on the pill causes less of these pain-producing substances to be released. Strangely, however, a few women, especially if underweight, actually complain of more menstrual cramping if they take some brands of pill—especially phasic ones. They may be helped by a single phase (monophasic) pill, and even more if it is 'tricycled' by running on the packets as explained on page 52. Indeed, another great advantage of the pill is:

2. *Ability to control the periods*. You have so much control that it is even possible, though not the normal routine, to take

the combined pill continuously and then have no vaginal bleeding at all. This is perfectly acceptable short term because of holidays and exams; and you can also as a 'once off' ploy take a few pills from a spare pack to make sure you never have periods at weekends, for instance. This is all discussed on pages 47–8, 53 (possible snags of tricycling); and 194–5 (re phasic pills, which have special rules).

3. *Mittelschmerz*. This word means 'middle pain' and refers to the pain of ovulation or egg-release. Quite a lot of women feel a slight ache in one or other groin at around the middle of the cycle, and some can use this to help them work out their 'safe period'. In some months in a few women it can be very severe. The pain is thought to be due to stretching of the rest of the ovary by the growing follicle at the middle of the cycle before it ruptures to release the egg (see Chapter 2): and when it does there may also be a small amount of painful internal bleeding. If the pain comes from the right ovary and is particularly severe, it can be very difficult to distinguish from appendicitis. Normal use of the pill prevents ovulation and so avoids both the regular monthly pain and this possibility of a mistaken diagnosis, which could even lead to an unnecessary operation.

4. *Pre-menstrual tension*. In the days leading up to the next period, many women are troubled by depression, irritability, feelings of bloatedness, weight gain, tenderness of the breasts, backache, headache, and other pains. These and other symptoms are often lumped together as the so-called 'pre-menstrual syndrome', or pre-menstrual 'tension'. Just how awful this makes this time of the month varies enormously from woman to woman, and from cycle to cycle in the same woman. But the symptoms can be quite incapacitating. It is more common for women to commit suicide, to have accidents, and to do less well than expected in exams at this time of the month than any other. Probably because the pill gives a constant dose of both types of hormone, oestrogen and progestogen, through the second half of the cycle, quite a lot of sufferers from pre-menstrual tension find it improved if they take the pill. However, some are not helped. And a few even complain of similar symptoms while taking the pill, particularly if it is a phasic pill (see page 194).

See pages 199–202 for how to handle abnormalities of the bleeding pattern produced by the pill.

The reproductive system: (b) Fertility and babies

Return of fertility after stopping the pill

From the beginning, doctors have been aware of the possibility that the pill, which acts by switching off the normal menstrual cycle, might delay its normal return. This might interfere with the ability of ex-pill-users to have babies when they wanted them. In fact every new year of research seems to reassure us more about this one. The Oxford/FPA study is particularly helpful. Among previously fertile women giving up contraception so as to conceive, by about 30 months those who stopped the pill were as likely to have had their next baby as ex-users of the IUD or the cap. But it did seem that ex-pill-users take up to 3–12 months longer to conceive. If the woman had never been pregnant before and was aged over 30, the higher figure (a year's extra delay) was more likely to apply. But even then there was nil to suggest that the pill could make anyone sterile.

There is a substantial minority of 10 to 15 per cent of women who, whatever previous method of family planning they have used, fail to get pregnant after trying for a baby for a year. This is the proportion of reduced fertility which is to be expected in any community. So if a woman stops the pill and fails to get pregnant, although it is very natural to blame the pill there is a better than 1 in 10 chance that it could be a coincidence.

Fertility also goes down with age. So sometimes the problem is partly connected with delaying too long before trying for a baby. This is a most important point. All methods of family planning share a common 'side-effect': they give modern women the freedom to delay starting their family, but this can sometimes be for a bit too long. Some women suffer from infertility at 35, yet could have conceived without difficulty at 20. Indeed a few have proved that by an earlier unplanned pregnancy. If possible (having found the right father!) try to start your family in your twenties or early thirties.

* A very few women, perhaps one in 200 who stop the pill,

develop amenorrhoea—absence of ovulation and periods—for over six months. The rate is the same among women whose partners stop using the condom, yet I have not heard it suggested that the condom could cause absent periods! Experts believe that in only a few if any such cases was the pill truly responsible, and even then only by bringing out a natural tendency. Usually the previous pill-use was a coincidence, and the regular substitute periods they were having on the pill were masking amenorrhoea which they would have had at that time if they were using another method. It has not been linked with any particular brand, has the same causes as when the pill has never been used, and can happen if the pill was used briefly or for a long time. Reassuringly, it is also now possible to treat this problem of no periods with almost 100 per cent success.

What about taking a routine break from the pill every two years or so to improve your fertility chances? Everything in the discussion above is against that being necessary, and see also pages 151 and 181. The 'bottom line' is that the pill is reversible, and *on stopping it women get back the fertility that nature gave them—for the age they have now reached*.

If you want to take breaks on health grounds there is another argument to consider on page 205.

Please note too that the problem of absent periods after stopping, or without ever having taken, the pill is a completely different one from absence of 'pill periods'. The latter means nothing at all in relation to your chances of having a baby in the future. In fact, those few women who have absent periods after stopping the pill very commonly had very regular 'periods'— hormone withdrawal bleeds—all the time that they were taking it. See pages 47–8, 199–202 for further discussion of this matter which many people find confusing.

Could the pill cause my next baby to be abnormal?

1. *After stopping the pill?* Provided it was discontinued well before conceiving, researchers have failed to detect any consistent increase—or decrease—in any type of abnormality. In 1980 there was a report about what are known as neural tube defects, or NTDs (a group of birth defects which include spina

bifida). It appeared that in South Wales there was an increased rate of NTDs among the offspring of women who conceived within three months of stopping the pill.

Researchers from South Wales and Leeds have also reported that if a woman had had a previous NTD baby, the risk of having another could be reduced if she took extra vitamins before and after the time of conception. If this means that NTDs are in part caused by low vitamin levels, and we know (page 89) that the pill lowers many of these, an ex-use effect of the pill looks possible.

All the same, other studies, before and since, especially a large one from Finland in 1981, have quite failed to show any link between NTDs or any other birth defect and recent use of the pill. Moreover an expert Scientific Group of the World Health Organization (WHO) declared quite simply in 1981 that there was *no evidence for any adverse effects on the fetus of pill-use prior to conception*—and this remains the view of WHO. Twin-births seem truly less common, however.

What then should you do if you are on the pill and want to stop it for a baby (page 77)? Those couples who are by nature extra cautious may, in addition, use a method like the sheath to arrange that two natural periods or three months go by before their planned baby is conceived. This has not been proved to help, though it should certainly do no harm. Although most experts think they are not important you may find it reassuring to know that the vitamin and mineral changes shown in Table 4 (page 88) should all be back to normal by then.

Should you take extra vitamins? I would advise you only to take extra vitamins in tablet form, either at this time *or after conception*, if so advised by your doctor. According to some of the research, the most relevant vitamin is probably folic acid, but there is plenty of this in any balanced diet. Good food sources include green vegetables, citrus fruits, lean meats, liver, kidney, and yeast extracts. A good diet is in fact the main thing.

Most importantly, *any woman who finds herself pregnant less than three months after stopping the pill should not be alarmed*. Literally millions of mothers have done this without any harm befalling their babies. Any extra risk is unproven, and if it exists it is clearly very, very small.

2. *What about pill-taking in early pregnancy?* The RCGP Study researchers have reported that 102 babies were born following pregnancies during which the pill continued to be taken for a while, usually by mistake. In the Oxford/FPA Study there were a further 66 such births. The rate of birth defects in these was no higher than would be expected in any group of women having a planned baby. But it seems that in these circumstances twinning is more likely (contrast with page 128).

This is most reassuring. Although 168 babies is not an enormous number, it must mean that any bad effect on unborn babies of the hormones used in current pills must be very infrequent. However, we cannot leave the story there. The articles published about unplanned pregnancy while taking the pill are many, but they are also contradictory and very confusing. To summarize things very briefly, it does seem that the high-dose artificial sex hormones which used to be taken by women to help to make the diagnosis of pregnancy could perhaps harm the baby. But now that there are perfectly safe and more accurate methods based on measuring the hormone hCG (page 37) in a sample of early morning urine, this outdated way of testing for pregnancy should never be used at all. These hormone pregnancy tests were rather different from the combined pill anyway, as they used much higher doses. Secondly, you may perhaps have heard the very disquieting story of the drug diethylstilboestrol (DES). This is even less relevant to the pill, as this particular variety of oestrogen— which has a quite different chemical formula—*never has been and never will be used in any combined contraceptive pills*. But the story does worry some people about the pill, so let us discuss it and learn its lessons here.

*   Shortly after the last war there was a vogue, particularly in America, to treat threatened miscarriage with DES, a synthetic oestrogen. It was later shown that the treatment made no difference to the outcome when bleeding occurred in early pregnancy. But the doctors concerned thought that at least no harm had been done to those babies who were born if the pregnancies did not miscarry. Tragically, however, although the girl babies who were born in these circumstances appeared entirely normal at birth, they proved much later on—as

teenagers—to be more likely to develop a form of cancer of the vagina that was previously almost unknown. If their mothers had been treated with this drug in pregnancy about one in 1,000 of these girls got this cancer. Other problems in the daughters, and even in the mothers, have been suggested by some researchers. Boys born following pregnancies treated with DES were also reported to be more likely to have various abnormalities of their urinary system or genital organs.

This sad story rams home the message, once again, that all except life-saving or proven safe drug treatment should be avoided during early pregnancy, particularly during the crucial first three months while all the organs of the baby are being formed.

What does this mean in practice? Even though there is no proof that *the pill* could harm a baby, it is surely best to play safe. You should never *start* taking contraceptives or any other hormones if you think you could already be pregnant. And if you think you might have become pregnant while taking the combined or progestogen-only pill, it is best to switch at once to another method until you know for sure one way or another. This is discussed in relation to missed or not-absorbed pills in Figures 11 (page 61) and 21 (page 212).

If pregnancy is confirmed, and you did take pills *after the conception*, it is you who must decide what, if anything, to do; though consultation with your partner and the doctor may help. Discuss whether any special tests should be done, such as detailed ultrasound scanning of the fetus. The increased risk of an abnormality is very small indeed, judging by those 168 babies mentioned earlier. This was also the view of that WHO Scientific Group (page 128). One estimate is *less than* one in 1,000. This is a low rate but I think it is definitely an overestimate for modern pills: especially as it came from studies which included babies born to mothers who took hormones other than for contraception, including that outdated pregnancy test using very high doses. Moreover, something not many people realize is that 20 in 1,000 of all babies have a serious birth defect. So a baby exposed to the pill's hormones during the first three months of pregnancy has an added risk which is much less than one-twentieth of the risk taken by all would-be parents.

The breasts

Breast enlargement

Some women say their breasts seem smaller, but far more users of the pill do notice their bust getting a little larger. The increase tends to reach its maximum by the second packet of pills, and not to continue afterwards. For most women and their partners, and in most cultures, this is seen as an advantage. Others may object. It occurs partly as a direct effect of the progestogen and oestrogen, but also because many pill-users have an increase in the blood level of one of their own hormones, prolactin. This is produced by the pituitary gland, and one of its effects is to stimulate the breasts.

* In fact, prolactin can occasionally do rather too good a job of breast stimulation, and lead to:

The appearance of milky fluid from the nipples

This unwanted secretion can be a nuisance and should always be mentioned to your doctor. This is because the level of the hormone prolactin ought to be measured, as, if it is particularly high, it could perhaps be coming from a pituitary adenoma, or microadenomas. These are tiny 'lumps', sometimes microscopic in size, formed in the pituitary gland. Such lumps can be treated very satisfactorily either medically or, rarely, by an operation. The pill does not cause them but, like pregnancy, it could make them enlarge and become more active if present. So if the pill is used in this rare condition, it should only be under expert supervision.

Tenderness of the breasts

This can be part of the whole range of symptoms of pre-menstrual tension, or it can occur alone. In some unfortunate women the tenderness can be so extreme that for a few days before each period they cannot bear their breasts being touched, even by clothing. If you have this problem (even if not quite as bad as that) you may be better off while on the pill. It is possible that you will not be helped; and a few women actually report the symptom for the first time on the pill, especially during the early months. There is an enormous amount of variation in how people respond to drugs, and the pill is no exception to that rule.

Benign breast disease

This general term is used to include a number of non-malignant problems of the breast which are sometimes called 'chronic mastitis', 'fibrocystic disease', and a variety of other names. They all refer to more or less generalized lumpiness of the breast which can be quite tender and vary from month to month and with the time of the month, usually worst just before a period. This is a definite plus point for the pill, as the usual microscopic type of this breast trouble tends to be less common during pill-use, especially long-term pill-use. Sometimes there is a definite lump which no surgeon can be sure is not cancer till he has removed it, and had it looked at under a microscope by a laboratory expert. As a result, quite often women have to be admitted for an operation, under general anaesthesia, to remove what is actually a benign breast lump. Yet this is the only safe way to handle the situation.

The point is that this chain of events is less likely in any woman who uses the pill. Here then is another kind of surgical operation that is statistically less likely if you are on the pill, which for this effect should be a fixed-dose type and preferably progestogen dominant (page 203). If you have had breast surgery, see page 142.

Once benign breast disease (BBD) is present it is a 'risk factor' for breast cancer. So there is a bit of a paradox here. On the one hand the pill reduces the risk of getting BBD in the first place. But on the other hand, doctors exercise extra caution if the breasts have the problem already, especially if a lump has had to be operated on. Established BBD is now seen as a so-called 'relative contra-indication' to using the pill. See pages 142, 184.

Interference with breast-feeding

The combined pill can quite commonly reduce the volume and quality of milk flow in women who are breast-feeding after recently having had a baby. It seems pointless to use the combined pill at this time, when the progestogen-only pill is available which does not interfere with the flow of milk (see Chapter 8). In combination with full breast-feeding the progestogen-only pill is close to 100 per cent effective. See also pages 138–42 for discussion of *breast cancer*.

Bones and joints

Premature closing of the epiphyses

There is a theoretical effect of oestrogen in the pill, that it might stop a young girl growing before she had achieved her full height. This is because, in animal research, oestrogen can affect the epiphyses (growing-points) of the long bones, to cause them to close prematurely. This does not occur with the tiny dose of oestrogen in modern pills, which after all contain progestogen as well. The pill should normally not be given until, at the earliest, menstrual cycles have become well and truly established, by which time a girl has almost reached her ultimate height. For some more relevant considerations in younger women, see pages 23–7, 28–31, 82, and 139.

Arthritis

Several groups of researchers suggested that women on the pill are less likely to suffer from one common troublesome variety known as rheumatoid arthritis. However, a Mayo Clinic Study from the USA in 1985 was unable to show this protective effect, which must therefore be quite small if present at all with modern pills. Yet if a woman has already got the disease it may be improved by the pill, as in pregnancy. Research continues. See also page 137.

Osteoporosis

This means thinning of the bones, making them more likely to fracture even without much trauma. It is a problem chiefly of women past the menopause. But it often begins earlier, in the years leading up to the final menstrual period, as the ovaries work less well. It can also affect younger women who are short of oestrogen from their own ovaries due to amenorrhoea (page 181), often connected with anorexia and weight loss, and some athletes. The problem can be prevented by the pill, as by hormone replacement therapy (HRT), due to the oestrogen it contains. Pill-takers have been found to reach the menopause with better bone density than other women—another useful benefit outside contraception.

So the pill can be of real value to older women who also want contraception (page 258). In younger cases at risk of osteoporosis, the pill is a valuable treatment, usually after special tests and under supervision from a hospital consultant.

The skin

Chloasma/melasma

These unusual words describe a fairly common brown discoloration which is mainly on the forehead and on each side of the face in front of the ears. It is obviously not a problem for black-skinned women, but can happen to other races in pregnancy (the 'pregnancy mask'), and to pill-users. It is usually first noticed when the weather is good. Some women also notice an increase of pigmentation in other parts of the body. Special sunscreen creams can be applied especially during the summer, and careful use of make-up when required may help.

Chloasma usually fades a little when the pill is stopped or, apparently, after transferring to the progestogen-only pill. It may not entirely disappear though, because of pigment having been actually laid down in the skin.

Photosensitivity (excessive sensitivity to sunlight)

This problem can affect women who have never been on the pill, but it is more common in those who have. Skin exposed to the sun's rays develops very itchy red weals (urticaria). Treatment for this is unsatisfactory and there may be only a slight improvement if the pill is stopped. It is fairly uncommon, but it may mean that the affected woman has to avoid sunbathing altogether. Very rarely it is an indication of one of the porphyrias (page 175).

Increase in facial or body hair (hirsutism)

This is fortunately very rare, especially with the modern low-dose pills, and nearly always has another cause (i.e. being on the pill is a coincidence). An oestrogen-dominant pill with one of the new progestogens may help, or Dianette (page 204). Dianette can be such a help that it is recommended to treat people with excessive hair growth who have no need of contraception. Extra hair may also have to be removed with the help of electrolysis or similar treatment from a skin specialist.

Loss of scalp hair

This can also occur in women who have never taken any sex hormones at all. In fact there was no suggestion in the RCGP Study that this might be caused by the pill. As after childbirth, however, it is reported that some women have a problem of excessive hair loss *after stopping* the pill. This corrects itself spontaneously, though full recovery of decent-length head hair could take a year or more.

Other skin diseases

A range of other skin troubles has been described, occurring for the first time or apparently being worsened in pill-users. Yet others are improved. They tend to have rather complicated names. Out of a long list, those which are probably or possibly promoted by the pill include: telangiectasia, rosacea, eczema, neurodermatitis, erythema nodosum, and erythema multiforme. Some of these may be linked to the problem of allergy (see page 137 for further discussion).

Herpes gestationis (which has nothing to do with the virus herpes) is another one. It is interesting because, like the form of jaundice mentioned on page 117, it can occur in pregnancy and is likely to recur or worsen if the same woman later goes on the pill.

Even added together these skin troubles are still quite uncommon. Rather than say more about them here, from the practical point of view you should take advice from your doctor if you ever develop any skin problem which you think might be due to or made worse by the pill.

Skin troubles often made better by the pill

1. *Acne.* The RCGP Study showed that this was particularly likely to be improved, but at the time all pills had 50 mcg or more of oestrogen in them. The story now seems a bit more complicated. Acne occurs chiefly because the tiny ducts or passages leading from the grease-producing glands of the skin, especially in the face and on the back, tend to get blocked. The oestrogen in the pill may help to stop this happening. Some women are simply unlucky in the actual grease-producing glands they have been given by nature, and just going on the pill may not be enough to help the situation. However, if your own acne is not improved or seems to be getting worse on the pill, it is worth asking to change to a more oestrogen-dominant brand (see page 204) using one of the new progestogens, or Dianette. There are also other treatments, and fortunately the problem does tend to improve with age.

2. *Hirsutism.* Oestrogen-dominant pills and Dianette can sometimes help this problem of unwanted hair growth too (page 204).

3. *Greasy hair.* This too may be helped by oestrogen-dominant pills.

4. *Wax in the ears.* The wax-producing glands of the ears are affected in rather the same way by the hormones of the pill as the grease-producing glands. As a result the RCGP Study also showed that you were less likely to have your ears syringed for wax in them!

*Anything else?

On top of everything mentioned elsewhere in these two chapters, there is some evidence, weaker in some cases than others, for the following collection of possible side-effects: the carpal tunnel syndrome, in which there is a gradual onset of tingling and pain in one or both hands; cramps and pains in the legs; gingivitis (inflammation of the gums); dry socket after tooth extraction; vertigo (dizziness); voice changes in singers; Raynaud's syndrome (excessive whitening and 'deadness' of the fingers in cold weather); and chilblains.

I have left till now two very important but more controversial subjects, about which there are still as many questions as answers.

*The body's immunity and allergy mechanism

The RCGP, Oxford/FPA, and Walnut Creek Studies all showed that pill-users were more likely than non-users to have various infections including chicken-pox, gastric flu, respiratory and urinary infections.

Other inflammations, of soft tissues or of the bowel (tenosynovitis, bursitis, synovitis, and Crohn's disease) have also been reported more commonly in pill-users.

These facts suggest that the pill can alter immunity. In addition, various skin troubles are often connected with allergy, and eczema, for instance, was twice as common in pill-users in the RCGP Study. Women can also develop an allergy, with specific antibodies (see page 237 for a further explanation of these), to either the progestogen or the oestrogen of the pill itself. This occurs even more rarely than with other commonly used drugs like penicillins, but can show itself by troublesome rashes or by painful swollen joints (polyarthritis). These clear up completely only when the pill is stopped, and would recur if the same hormone were to be given again. So allergies to the pill itself certainly occur. Whether allergies to other substances happen more readily because the pill is being taken is not so clear, though the increased rate of hay fever is suggestive (page 115).

Another possibility is allergy to a person's own tissues causing so-called auto-immune diseases. It does appear that the pill can sometimes aggravate the symptoms and signs of one of these, systemic lupus erythematosus (SLE), which affects connective tissues in the body. Thrombosis is more likely in SLE so the pill is best avoided if it is diagnosed.

The number of white cells in the blood is increased in pill-users, and experiments on the ones called lymphocytes—which are much involved in this immune/allergy system—have shown that the pill can alter their activities.

The immune/allergy system is involved in causing several

types of thyroid disease and arthritis. As the pill seems to have possible protective effects (pages 90 and 133), perhaps some good effects too are due to an alteration in this system, caused by the pill's hormones.

What about cancer?

The pill does contain powerful hormones, and hormones have been shown to affect the growth of some cancers, in animals and in humans. So ever since the pill was first marketed there has always been the possibility that it might be found to increase the risk of some type of cancer. Secondly, it is one of the best-known facts of cancer research that cancers may not develop until after many years—up to 30 years—of exposure to any cancer-producing agent. The pill has been around for only about that time. We are therefore only now beginning to obtain useful information about possible links between it and some forms of cancer. Although in many cases these have not yet been confirmed, in view of the widespread nature of the pill's effects we should not be too surprised if it can in fact modify the risk of getting certain cancers. The important thing is that it operates either way: promoting some but actually reducing the likelihood of other types. Two examples of cancers which are now proven to be less frequent in pill-takers than other women are those which start in the endometrium and ovary (see below).

So it begins to look (see on a few pages if you like, to Figure 15) a bit like 'swings and roundabouts', with the good effects tending to balance the bad. *The overall risk of cancer in pill-takers may stay about the same* as that for the general population. But this is an unfolding story, which will not be fully told for some time yet.

*The breast

In the United States, it seems that one in every 11 women will develop breast cancer at some time in her life. Many will eventually die, years later, of something quite different. And the rate is not quite as high in other developed countries, such as Britain. But if the pill were found to cause any change in the frequency of this disease—either way—it would be enormously important.

During the last 30 years the pill has increasingly been used, and breast cancer rates have increased in many countries. It is tempting to conclude that the pill is to blame. If that were so, it is odd that the statistics show a rise in all age-groups, and the greatest rise among older women who never had a chance to take the pill. Moreover there have been many other relevant changes in society during the same 30 years: in diet for a start, plus increased rates of several known risk factors. These are:

- Younger ages at the first menstrual period.
- Later ages at the menopause.
- More women delaying the birth of their first child, to after age 30. (This is known to increase breast-cancer rates whatever method of family planning is used.)
- More women not breast-feeding their babies (preferably for many months). Breast-feeding is *protective*.
- The family history of a close relative (mother or sister) with breast cancer, especially if it was diagnosed under age 45 (page 141).
- Benign breast disease (page 132).
- Possibly, eating high fat diets.

Unhelpfully, the research in this field is copious, complicated, confusing, and often contradictory! One thing that is clear, though, is that *taking the pill between about the ages of 25 and 45 does not increase the risk*. But taking it when young, before the woman's first baby is born, is more of a problem.

* An accepted summing-up of all the research to date is: There is *probably*, not certainly since it is not confirmed by the cancer registration statistics, an increased risk of breast cancer occurring at a young age (defined as under about age 35); but if so it probably diminishes or disappears at older ages. Remotely, the risk might yet be found to persist to later ages.

At the time of writing, the research which gives us the main lead is what is known as the UK National Case-Control (UKNCC) Study (1989). They reported an increase in the risk, from a normal rate of 1 in 500 in the relevant age-group, to 1 in 350 if the pill had been used for four or more years.

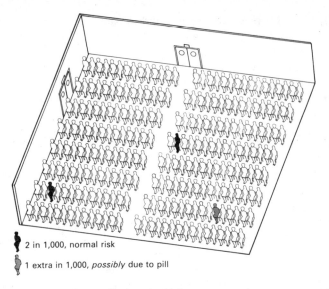

 2 in 1,000, normal risk

1 extra in 1,000, *possibly* due to pill

Fig. 14 Chance of being diagnosed with breast cancer, in young women aged 35 or less

What does this really mean? Imagine (Figure 14) a concert hall packed with 1,000 young women, all no older than 35 years. It is a fact that *two* of them, sitting on those chairs, will be under treatment currently for breast cancer. (That is what the normal rate of 1 in 500 means). Now imagine everyone leaving and a new audience troops in: 1,000 women of the same ages (35 years and younger), but this time all have taken the pill for at least four years. Now there will be *three* under treatment. Two of them cannot blame the pill, since there were two in the first audience.

So the conclusion is that only one in 1,000 pill-takers would develop breast cancer *because of* the pill. What is more, it is believed that she is someone who was destined to get it later, say at 45, anyway. The pill may in fact be 'bringing out' a cancer already on board (acting as what is known as a co-factor).

This is still hardly good news. But many women with whom I have used the illustration above have told me that the effectiveness and convenience of the pill and all its other benefits (which include protection against other cancers) simply outweigh this problem, for them.

What now, in practice?

1. First the *whole* cancer story (not forgetting the good news which follows) needs now to be discussed as part of routine pill counselling with all young pill-takers before they start, or at some appropriate time in the first four years of use.

2. If the pill really does increase breast cancer risk in younger women, it is likely this will be minimized by using modern pill brands which cause least disturbance to body chemistry. The new progestogens *might* be better than the older ones, norethisterone or levonorgestrel (page 154), though it is too soon to be sure. The UKNCC Study definitely showed that the low-oestrogen pills seemed to have the least risk. Fortunately these are precisely the same ones which are recommended to reduce the risk of circulatory disease (page 189). It remains acceptable for doctors to supply such pills with no arbitrary time limit to young people, even teenagers. This practice is supported by the UK Committee on the Safety of Medicines.

However Loestrin 20 and Mercilon, pages 191–2, are *not* usually ideal for teenagers, since they have too small a margin for pill-taking errors and the rate of 'breakthrough' bleeding tends to be unacceptable.

3. What if *there is a close family history of breast cancer (as defined above)*?

This roughly doubles the risk. But according to research, the pill adds no more to the risk problem such women already have than (if the UKNCC Study is true) would be added by the pill to an ordinary young woman. Thus the *extra increment* of risk seems to be the same. After explaining this, *some* will be happy to take that same extra possible risk as anyone else takes. *Others* may say they would rather not take the chance of adding anything to what risk they already have (and cannot change)— and so would prefer to use another method. This must be their decision after discussion of all known facts.

In short, the family history is now called a *relative contra-indication*. This means the pill *may* be used, for perhaps a more limited duration than usual, with extra counselling about the pros and cons and then careful supervision.

4. What if *the woman has benign breast disease*? (Page 132.)

This is again a relative contra-indication, with no known *extra* increment of risk due to the pill: similar in many ways to the family history situation above. If you are seeing a surgeon for a problem with your breasts, ask for his expert opinion as to whether it is advisable to continue with or start taking the pill.

If you had an earlier operation for a lump in the breast, find out if it showed in the laboratory any tissue with what is called epithelial atypia (abnormal cells). *In that unusual case the pill really would be best avoided altogether.* Similarly if a woman actually has had breast cancer treated, she should stop or avoid the pill and all sex hormones except as part of treatment recommended by the doctor looking after her for the disease.

5. Whether or not they have ever taken the pill, and especially if any of the above risk factors apply, all women should examine their own breasts regularly each month. This is best done after periods, using the flat of the extended fingers. This is just common sense, and if you are in any doubt about how to do it you should ask to be taught by your doctor or nurse, with the help of an illustrated leaflet.

6. All women, especially those with a positive family history, should breastfeed any babies they have as long as they can (page 139).

*The uterus: (a) the cervix (entrance to the womb)

A report in 1983 from the Oxford/FPA Study (page 104) suggested increased rates of this cancer, and of the pre-cancer changes picked up by cervical smears, with increasing duration of use of the pill. After more than eight years the maximum rate was 2–3 times that in non-users (actually IUD-users). Another researcher also reported in 1977 that the pill seemed to accelerate the slow rate at which the earliest changes can sometimes progress to actual cancer, though other workers have not found this effect.

Cancer of the cervix is really a sexually transmitted disease (page 28). It is caused most probably by a virus or a combination of viruses transmitted sexually. Hence barrier methods like the diaphragm are protective. The risk for someone with many sexual partners can be many times that of a one-man woman whose partner is a one-woman man. *Smoking* also much increases the risk of this cancer, and its pre-cancer stages shown on cervical smears. Even if we accept—not every expert does—the Oxford report and some others since which point a finger at the pill, cigarettes and sexual life-style (of self or partner(s)) are much more important factors. At worst the pill is seen as a weak co-factor. It is never the cause of the cancer but is perhaps able to promote the abnormal cell changes once they have been started.

In practice, the main point is that pill-users should have regular cervical smears which should catch the earliest abnormalities in plenty of time for preventive treatment. How often, for pill-takers especially if they also smoke? This is disputed, but I would say 3-yearly anyway or 2-yearly where resources permit; and annually if there are the risk factors on page 28 or abnormal cells have been found.

May you stay on the pill if you have or have had an abnormal smear? The short answer is 'yes'. I consider that abnormal smears are only a weak relative contra-indication (see above and page 184). Mild cell changes commonly resolve naturally, so the smear may just be repeated every few months. Or the abnormality may need to be removed, using colposcopy (which is a special telescope magnifier for examining the cervix) and various techniques like the laser or other minor surgery. But if after full discussion of all the facts, and the question marks, you prefer the pill to any of the alternatives, your choice should be respected. It will of course be vital to have smear tests more often than usual, as ordered by your gynaecologist, and probably for the rest of your life—whether you take the pill or not.

* (b) The endometrium (lining of the womb)

Researchers from an excellent American study, known as the CASH (Cancer and Sex Hormones) Study, have shown a halving of the risk if the pill is taken for at least one year, and a threefold reduction after five years. This *protective effect* has been confirmed by at least six other studies, and encouragingly seems to persist in ex-users—for 15 years, possibly even longer.

* Cancer of this type was more likely to occur in women who

used the high-oestrogen so-called 'sequential' pills—but these have not been prescribed in the UK for more than 20 years.

* The ovary

At least nine studies report a clear-cut protective effect which is greater the longer the pill has been used. This is really important, since this cancer kills more than any other gynaeco-logical malignancy. After five years the CASH Study reports a threefold reduction in the risk, and protection continues among ex-users for at least 15 years, maybe even for life.

It is probably not coincidental that both the last two cancers are beneficially affected by the pill: both are commoner in those women who have had many menstrual cycles. This is an unnatural state of affairs (see pages 49–51) which is avoided by pill-takers who do not have *true* periods at all. They therefore seem to share some of the health advantages of women who have many pregnancies.

* Trophoblastic disease

Here there is complete failure of the normal development of a pregnancy. It is not itself a cancer, but it has a very small risk of turning into one. No embryo develops, and the afterbirth fills the uterus to make it seem like a bag full of very mushy grapes. These produce large amounts of the special pregnancy hormone hCG (see page 37). Sooner or later, as this is never going to be a successful pregnancy, bleeding occurs. Eventually the uterus has to be emptied under anaesthetic in hospital, by a D & C.

Subsequently, the patient has to be very carefully followed up. The main thing that has to be done during follow-up is a regular special blood or urine test to measure the hCG level. In Britain these tests are mailed to specific Regional Centres. In nearly all patients, the level falls steadily to nil in a few months, and that is really the end of the story. In a tiny minority, however, the level of hCG stays up, and this means that powerful drugs must be given as it is due to the very beginnings of a cancer called *choriocarcinoma*. If this is treated early the outcome is almost always complete cure.

The pill does not make the original trophoblastic disease more likely to happen, but it comes into the story here. Researchers in London have shown that if the pill is taken before the hCG level in the blood has declined to zero, the chances of needing the powerful drug treatment for the early cancer are about doubled. Other research workers have failed to confirm this, however, and in the USA supervised use of the pill is allowed even when the hCG level is high.

In my view until the uncertainty is resolved, both combined and progestogen-only pills—and injectables (page 255)—are best avoided altogether by a woman who has had this unusual trouble. This makes it an *absolute* or (strong) *relative contra-indication* to the pill, see page 176—but only until she is informed that her hCG test is back to normal. After discussion with her gynaecologist or other doctor, oral contraception could then be considered once again as an option.

*Melanoma

This cancer can develop from a mole, one of those black patches which people have on their skin. Almost everyone has a few of these. The change to cancer is more likely in skin exposed to a lot of sunlight. In areas like California and Australia where there is a lot of sun it seemed possible in some studies, but not in others, that the pill might slightly increase the chances of the transformation of an ordinary mole into this cancer. But as there is a distinct possibility that pill-users in the research populations may have sunbathed more than non-users, it seems likely at the time of writing (1991) that the pill does not promote this cancer.

*Liver

The pill may promote primary liver cancer, an exceedingly rare disease (in the UK <1 case per 100,000 long-term pill-users). Tumours of a non-cancerous kind are certainly linked with long-term use. They too are very rare. They appear as lumps on the liver. Since they contain a great many blood-vessels they can sometimes cause dangerous internal bleeding—leading to an emergency operation to stop this and remove the tumour.

Professor Martin Vessey is in charge of the Oxford/FPA study (page 104). Using the best data available he performed a computer analysis, which was published by the Royal Society of Medicine in 1990. He compared the cancer deaths to be expected among one million women using the pill with those among another million women who were partners of condom-users, both populations starting at age 16 and then relying on sterilization after age 35. By the time they were 50, the computer actually found it likely that there would be more cancer deaths (chiefly 1,400 deaths from cancer of the ovary) among the condom-using million than among the ever-users of the pill! See Figure 15.

To conclude, if all the 'pros' and 'cons' are carefully weighed up, the evidence so far does not disprove the following statement:

The average informed pill-user may continue to take modern ultra-low-dose pills without fearing any increase in her OVERALL cancer risk.

But, how long is it safe to continue? See pages 149–52. And remember, the situation is constantly under review, as new facts emerge.

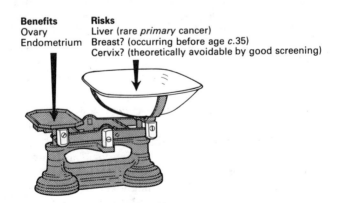

Benefits   **Risks**
Ovary   Liver (rare *primary* cancer)
Endometrium   Breast? (occurring before age *c*.35)
                   Cervix? (theoretically avoidable by good screening)

Fig. 15 Cancer and the pill: a balance

*How reliable are the research studies on the pill?

Although they are the best available, we do have to be a little cautious when applying the results of research like the RCGP, Walnut Creek, and Oxford/FPA Studies. For a start, there are differences between the sort of women who use a method like the pill and those who do not. These differences could lead to any trouble or apparent benefit which arises being put down to the pill when it was really connected with some other feature of the woman herself. In general, pill-users seem to be generally healthier than non-users, rather than the reverse.

Secondly, in the RCGP and Walnut Creek studies, though not in the Oxford/FPA one, the pill-users went more often to their doctors as a routine, to collect their prescriptions. While there, they could be more likely to mention a problem they had noticed than the non-pill-users with whom they were compared, who would have to make a special visit. As the research workers are aware of this possible bias attempts have been made to allow for it.

Thirdly, most studies omit teenagers, and use of modern pills (pages 139, 164).

What about the risks of the pill in less developed countries?

These have been inadequately examined so far. The research has nearly all been done in 'over-developed' countries, where diseases of the circulation such as heart attacks and strokes in relatively young people are commoner than in developing countries. This is probably because there are so many things wrong with the diet, combined with the popularity of smoking and the unpopularity of exercise, among other things. This would suggest that use of the pill should be even more reasonable for women in the less developed countries; particularly in comparison with the tragically high rate of death and serious complications of pregnancy and childbirth in the absence of good medical care, which many of them have to face (see Figure 1, page 6).

A special advantage of the pill is connected with anaemia of the type due to shortage of iron, which is more common because of malnutrition and conditions such as worms. The pill reduces both blood loss at periods and loss of iron to the baby in repeated pregnancies. On the other hand, the pill has effects on vitamins (see Table 4 on page 88, and page 90). Recent research suggests that extra vitamins are helpful for women with dietary deficiencies—but not for healthy pill-users anywhere.

Research in developing countries by international bodies such as the World Health Organization (WHO) is now showing some differences in body chemistry. Pill-users in Dublin get more of the changes favouring blood-clotting than women in Salvador (Brazil) taking the same brand. And, according to some researchers, poor nutrition and reduced amounts of body fat may lower the blood levels of the pill's hormones after taking standard pills. Thus, underweight, malnourished women may, paradoxically, be at extra risk of pregnancy, and probably should not take the very lowest-dose pills. Another factor which favours slightly higher-dose pills is the observation that erratic pill-taking is rather common among women in developing countries (depending very much on how well they have been taught).

We just do not know how important differences between women in the less developed countries and those who have been studied in the 'over-developed' world may be. Differences might be expected due to heredity: for example, there could be as yet undiscovered racial differences in body chemistry, leading to different handling of the pill's hormones by the body. The effects that being on the pill might have in women suffering from the various chronic tropical diseases are still being studied, including: malaria; leprosy; liver fluke infection; and bilharzia. WHO has reported a possible slight increase in activity of the parasites among pill-users with bilharzia. But the pill had no harmful effects on tests of liver function in this disease.

More research is needed. But so far no reports have identified any definite extra risk for pill-users in developing countries compared with those in Europe and North America. Everything points instead to the benefits being even greater.

*What are the long-term or long-delayed effects of taking the pill?

For an individual woman, this question needs to be broken down to three different but closely connected questions:

1. *How long should one continue taking the pill?*

2. *Should one take breaks* every two years or every five years?

3. Irrespective of the answers to questions 1 and 2, *what is the upper age limit for continuing to take the pill*?

From the point of view of preserving future fertility, the answer is clear to all these questions. There is no connection between fertility problems and how long the pill was previously used, in total, with or without breaks. Routine breaks at any set time-interval are therefore illogical (page 127). The combined pill seems to be truly a reversible method of contraception. And the upper age limit for the best chance of success when it comes to trying for a baby is the same, whether discontinuing the pill or any other method: *if circumstances permit, try to start your family in your twenties or early thirties*.

*Side-effects

Most of the risks (and benefits) seem to apply primarily while the pill is actually being taken. And if the pill is stopped, things seem to return to normal within a few weeks. These statements apply to the studies of body chemistry which were described earlier (page 90, and Table 4, page 88); to the risk of many of the serious side-effects such as venous thrombosis, and of the less serious but annoying ones such as weight gain and headaches; and of course to the beneficial effects on the menstrual cycle.

*Long-term use and diseases of the circulation

As stated on page 104, the RCGP Study now shows no detectable increase in the overall risk with increasing duration of use in current users. However, in a later report (1983), the researchers were more doubtful about the absence of a duration-of-use effect for individual diseases, particularly stroke.

It has also been shown before that raised blood pressure is diagnosed increasingly often, the longer the pill has been used. No duration-of-use effect has yet been found for other conditions such as heart attack or venous thrombosis.

*Possible residual effects in ex-users

A large study (1988) in America following up nurses who were ex-takers of the pill has failed to show any increased risk of circulatory diseases compared with never-users. This is reassuring and suggests that an earlier American study reported in the last edition of *The Pill* was incorrect.

However the increased risk of strokes does appear from the RCGP research to continue in ex-users, for more than six years after the pill was last taken. It is important to remember that strokes are extremely rare in young women; the risk appears to be focused on those with other risk factors (pages 97–8), especially smoking; and it is probably also at a lower level than in current users.

How then do we minimize the risk of diseases of the circulation?

Age? This question among those which began this section was partly answered on pages 105–7. Smokers should consider stopping at age 30 and must transfer to another method at the age of 35. For others the situation has changed from the last edition, since that most important statement by the relevant FDA Medical Advisory Committee on 26 October 1989. They recommended:

> *The removal of all age limits on the use of (combined) oral contraceptives by healthy non-smoking women* (i.e. completely without risk factors, page 97).

This means that in such women the appropriate pill brands may on their request be used right up to the menopause . . . The reasons for this quite dramatic change in policy are: we now know the pill's risks although they are greater in older women, are much less than used to be thought for those without risk factors; we know more about the benefits as women get older, especially protection against gynaecological problems like ultra-heavy periods leading to the risks of hysterectomy; and we are now able to use much safer pills (pages 189–92).

Breaks? We can, I think, give a definite answer 'no' to the question about taking breaks every two or every 10 years. One way of looking at this is: because you only take the pill for three weeks in four, if you have been on it for 10 years you have really only taken it for seven and a half years. What is more you have already taken 130 breaks: how many more do you want? Those breaks really do seem to help. Various fascinating studies of body chemistry have now reported that certain abnormal measurements on pill treatment return towards normal during the pill-free interval of (normally) seven days. So the breaks are beginning to appear important as a time of 'rest' for the system, when the body adjusts before the next three weeks of pill-taking. See also page 52 re tricycling.

There is no research to suggest that taking additional breaks over and above those regular ones would reduce overall risks, unless the breaks were long enough to have a definite impact on the *total accumulated duration* of use. In other words, suppose a pill-user decides to take a 6-month break every two years: after 12 years she will have accumulated 10 years of use, without, so far as we know, lessening her risk as compared with someone who took the pill continuously for 10 years. In short, *repeated breaks from pill-taking are a nuisance, are of no proven benefit, and also have been known to lead to unplanned pregnancies . . .*

Duration? As far as the circulation is concerned, this issue might first be faced and discussed after 10 years' accumulated use (with or without breaks). Smokers should consider 15 years as the absolute maximum, provided they are also under 35 and have normal blood pressure. Non-smokers who are free of risk factors and using modern 'lipid-friendly brands' (pages 155–6) no longer need consider that there is any fixed upper limit on circulatory disease grounds—such as 20 years' use, as was previously suggested. They may well not wish to go on for so long, but if they do they may now be permitted to do so.

Cancer and duration of use/ex-use

Please read pages 138–46, if you have not already done so. If the pill is finally proved to increase the risk of any important cancer—not so, as yet—the harmful effect could be greater the longer the pill were used, and might persist to some extent in ex-users. If the pill reduces a risk, as it does for cancer of the ovary and endometrium, the protective effect is certainly greater the longer the duration of use, and continues among ex-users.

Once again—see pages 138, 146—we have 'swings and round-abouts': good effects of long-term pill-use tending to balance the bad. As above, breaks are unlikely to help unless they are long ones, as the evidence points to total duration. But there are more question marks about long-term use by the young. So far the evidence about breast cancer (pages 138–42) does not support setting an arbitrary limit to the number of years' use by women under say age 25 or before their first baby—unless they are at special risk (pages 141–2). In that case four or five years might be the recommended maximum while we wait for more data.

In conclusion, nothing stated here overrides the importance of your own views and intuition. By all means take short-term or longer breaks if this helps your own peace of mind. But do be careful in your use of another method, without gambling!—unless you really want a baby.

*What do the changes in body chemistry mean?

See Table 4 (pages 88–9). A wide variety of changes have been described in the blood of pill-users, and often their meaning from the point of view of the health of the person concerned is completely unknown. Some of them must be connected in some way with known unwanted effects of the pill: for instance, the changes in blood lipids and clotting factors. Even here the full details of the connection between the blood changes and the appearance of symptoms are not fully worked out. The majority of the remainder seem harmless, but only time and a lot more research will prove if this is so.

One of the main aims of research into body chemistry is to find a simple and accurate test of a body fluid such as blood or, preferably, saliva or urine, which would identify those women who should not be on the pill because they are at too high a risk of trouble. A lot can already be done to avoid giving the pill to women at special risk (see page 171). Tests on blood and other fluids, however, have so far been disappointing; blood lipid (fat) studies for example are very complicated and even the experts may not be sure what they mean in any individual. They are not suitable as so-called 'screening' tests and have to be reserved primarily for women who have a family history suggesting that they might prove to be abnormal.

Of course, there is already one quite useful test: the blood pressure of pill-users. Stopping the pill when this becomes raised may prevent a stroke from occurring (page 100) and may perhaps protect the pill-user from other circulatory troubles too (pages 102–3).

Are there differences between the different brands of pill?

The short answer is 'yes, but we do not know for sure which is the "best buy"'. There are many different varieties of pill, including progestogen-only pills, on the British market, and other formulations also are used in other countries. Two different oestrogens are used and several different progestogens, in varying combinations. The currently available British ones are shown in Tables 9, 10, and 12 (pages 186–7, 188, 221). As the next section explains, low-dose brands from Table 9 are now preferred. They all use the same oestrogen (ethinyloestradiol).

*How much safer are the modern very low-oestrogen pills? and the progestogen-only pills?

Although we cannot distinguish between individual brands, research is available that strongly suggests that, as far as risk is concerned, the lower the dose of artificial hormone taken, the better: and the amount of hormones in pills taken for contraception has diminished most dramatically since they were first introduced. Table 5 shows how among the modern ultra-low-dose combined pills, which are still highly effective against pregnancy, it is possible to use more than 7 times less oestrogen. And as much of the same progestogen used to be taken in one day, in Enovid 10, as is now taken in one month!

Table 5 Reduction in hormone dose given since combined pills were first introduced

	Amount used then (1960–2)	*Minimum* of same hormone used now (1991)
Dose of oestrogen (ethinyloestradiol)	150 mcg in Enovid 10	20 mcg in Mercilon or Loestrin 20
Dose of progestogen (norethisterone)	10000 mcg in Ortho-novum 10	500 mcg in { Ovysmen Brevinor

It seems now that the old idea that oestrogen was the main hormone causing unwanted effects is too simple. *Oestrogen* is certainly the hormone that causes the main changes in clotting factors, predisposing to thrombosis in veins but also in arteries if there is any atherosclerosis (pages 96–7). Researchers then studied women taking different brands containing the same oestrogen dose, but with varying doses of either norethisterone (NET) or levonorgestrel (LNG). Those were the standard progestogens in use until the new, more 'selective' ones (desogestrel and gestodene) came along. Certain conditions were found to become more frequent as the dose of those progestogens increased, suggesting that the progestogen was important in causing the problem. A good example is blood pressure: the rate of diagnosis of high blood pressure (hypertension) was greatest in the pill with the highest dose of NET progestogen, least in the one with the lowest dose, as shown in Table 6. The dose of ethinyloestradiol is the same in all three pills (50 mcg).

Research reported in the early 1980s suggests that arterial diseases, especially heart attacks and strokes, are related in a similar way to increasing NET or LNG progestogen dose. Other examples of this are gallstones, acne, and thrombosis in superficial veins of the leg. It also appears that progestogens of the NET/LNG type have important effects on body chemistry. This includes a lowering of one component of the blood lipids, high-density lipoprotein-cholesterol (HDL-2-cholesterol). Many

Table 6 Blood pressure according to dose of progestogen (RCGP Study)

Dose (micrograms) of progestogen (norethisterone acetate, NET-type)	Rate of diagnosis of high blood pressure
4000	13.9 per 1,000 women per year
3000	12.3　　　　　"
1000	8.2　　　　　"

experts think this substance is protective, so to reduce it may increase the risk of diseases of the circulation.

Blood glucose and insulin levels (especially the latter) tend also to be raised by a high content of NET or LNG progestogen. These changes imitate mild diabetes which is linked with an increased risk of atherosclerosis (page 172)—not that we can be sure this would be true when caused in a different way by the pill. But it is a further reason for concern to reduce the progestogenic as well as the oestrogenic strength of the formulations used. See page 188 re the suspect brands.

It seems clear for least effect on body chemistry, and *probably* also for lowest health risk, the minimum of both hormones should be used. This is how to give effect to that working rule we highlighted on page 87.

Just reducing the dose was not satisfactory. Things are not that simple. As lower and lower doses were tried, following the above reasoning, so there were more complaints about *irregular (breakthrough) bleeding*. The first answer (in the late 1970s) was to introduce variable-dose, so-called phasic pills (described on pages 192–6). They reduced the LNG or NET progestogen as well as the oestrogen to a minimum, yet at the same time they gave most women an acceptable pattern of bleeding and remained effective at preventing pregnancy.

A more recent solution has been the introduction in the 1980s of the new 'selective' progestogens, the first two examples of which are desogestrel (as in Marvelon and Mercilon) and gestodene (used in Femodene/Minulet). 'Selective' means that they give more of what we want, which is contraception and a strong effect to control bleeding from the uterus, and less of what we do not want, namely unwanted effects on blood fats (lipids). This is why I call them 'lipid-friendly'. Pills using these progestogens are becoming more and more popular, as they are low dose, producing less apparently bad changes in body chemistry, and yet without unacceptable bleeding or the need to use phasic packaging.

Good effects may also depend on the progestogen. The reduction in the rate of benign breast disease mentioned on page 132, and the protective effect against symptoms, chiefly bleeding, from fibroids (page 121) have both been found to be greater the greater the progestogen content of the pill being given. Progestogen also appears to be linked with the reduced risk of pelvic infection (page 120) and of cancer of the endometrium (page 143).

Progestogen-only pills (POPs), which are considered in Chapter 8, not only have no oestrogen, but also have less progestogen than most combined pills. So they ought by rights to have the lowest health risk of all, though too little research has yet been done to be quite sure about this (see pages 207, 217).

To sum up, the best advice for most pill-users is to request a pill brand from among those giving the lowest known '*body impact*' (which is more important than simply *dose*) of both hormones. This policy not only reduces the risk of arterial and venous diseases in older women and possibly breast cancer in young women (see page 141); it also lessens the frequency of those so-called 'minor' side-effects listed on page 75. Higher doses should be reserved for the few exceptions: chiefly, problems with bleeding (see pages 199–201) and the long-term use of enzyme-inducing drugs (page 71).

6

....

The pill in perspective

Table 7 is a summary of most of the effects for which there is at least some evidence of a link with the pill. It is, of necessity, not entirely comprehensive. The emphasis to be given to any one effect depends on the answers to four important questions:

1. *How strong is the evidence?* Has it been consistently shown by more than one group of researchers? And/or is there a reason for expecting the effect, such as a known change in body chemistry?

2. *How important is the condition being caused, worsened, or improved?*

3. *How large is the effect of the pill? (How many times more or less common is the condition in pill-users?)*

4. *How common is the condition anyway?*

Questions 3 and 4 are linked in the way to be described on page 163 (attributable risk), and they all apply to the good as well as the bad effects, of course. At the end of the day the conclusion, based on the answer to all four, depends on the individual judgement of the informed person, whether doctor or pill-user. Try answering these questions: which is the more important in deciding about the pill today, some very preliminary and unconfirmed evidence that the pill might increase the chance of a severe allergy in a tiny number of women? Or the certainty that abnormal pigmentation (chloasma) will develop in a larger number? And how do you match either with the certainty that an even larger number of pill-users will not get the iron deficiency anaemia due to heavy periods which they would otherwise suffer?

Although the actual amount of the extra risk or benefit may be hotly debated, the evidence linking them with the pill to

Table 7 Side-effects of the combined pill

Good Effects	
Common	**Uncommon or rare**
• (Acne—less with some pills)	• Bones—prevents osteoporosis
• Benign breast disease—less	• Cancer of ovary—less
• Breast tenderness—usually less	• Cancer of endometrium—less
• Effective—nearly 100 per cent (hence relief of *fear* of pregnancy)	• (Duodenal ulcers—? less)
	• Ectopic pregnancies—much less
• Good social effects (pages 18–20)	• Endometriosis—less
• Intercourse—unaffected by the method	• Fibroids—fewer troubles
	• Ovarian cysts—less
	• (Rheumatoid arthritis—?? less)
	• (Thyroid disease—? less)
	• (Toxic shock—? less)

Menstrual cycle improved:
- More regular bleeding
- Timing of 'periods' can be controlled (pages 50, 124–5)
- No ovulation pain
- (Less pre-menstrual tension)
- Less period pain
- Less heavy bleeding, therefore:
- Less anaemia
- Pelvic infection—less
- Poisoning—almost impossible
- Reversible—nearly 100 per cent
- (Trichomonas vaginitis—? less)
- (Unwanted hair growth—less with some pills)
- Wax in the ears—less, overall

some extent is at least adequate for the majority of the conditions mentioned in the last two chapters. In Table 7 those side-effects about which the evidence is weakest, or where the net effect of the pill is uncertain, are in brackets. There is no doubt that some women report loss of libido on the pill, for instance, but others report improvement: so loss of libido is in brackets because it is difficult to be sure what the net (overall) effect would be in a large group of pill-users.

Figure 16 shows somewhat more clearly, because the facts are known from the RCGP Study, how frequent certain of the good

Bad Effects

Common	Uncommon or rare
• Absent bleeding in pill-free week	• Breast pain
• (Allergies)	• (Cancer of breast—in young)
• Bleeding on pill-taking days	• (Cancer of cervix—? co-factor)
• Breast enlargement*	• Chloasma or other skin troubles
• Cramps and pains in legs, or in arms	• Crohn's disease
• Cystitis and other urinary infections	• Contact lens troubles
• (Depression)	• Delayed return of fertility
• Ectopy of cervix with increased vaginal discharge	• Eye troubles
• Fluid retention/bloatedness	• Fibroids—rarely enlargement and pain
• Gum inflammation	• Gallstones
• Headaches	• Heart attacks
• (Loss of libido)	• Hypertension
• Migraine	• Jaundice
• Nausea	• Milky fluid from breasts
• Reduced resistance to some infections	• Phlebitis (thrombosis of superficial veins)
• Unwanted social side-effects (pages 23–30)	• Strokes
• Weight gain*	• Tumours of liver (adenoma and very rare primary cancer)
	• Venous thrombosis with or without pulmonary embolism

Notes: 1. The order is alphabetical in each list. The various effects obviously vary enormously in their relative importance.

2. ?'s and brackets round an item mean conflicting research so that doubt remains about whether, or to what extent, the pill causes the effect. Brackets on their own mean the pill can have real but quite opposite effects in different women: e.g. some pill-takers report *increased* pre-menstrual tension, others *increased* libido, allergies can improve or worsen.

3. * These may seem good effects to some underweight women.

and bad effects are, and by how much the pill increases or reduces their rate of occurrence.

If you have read right through the last two chapters, you are now perhaps overwhelmed by the number and variety of non-contraceptive effects of the pill. You may well be wondering how anyone can bring herself to use it. But suppose that you had instead been reading a very comprehensive account by a Casualty Surgeon of all the injuries and long-term complications which have been linked with road accidents—would you not

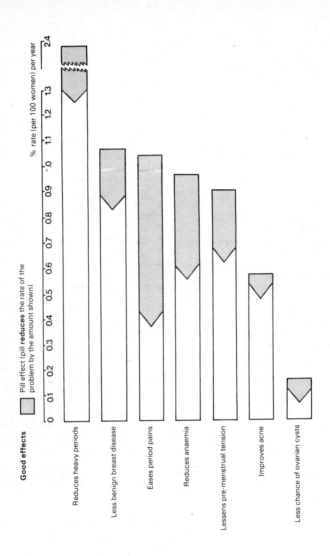

Good effects

Pill effect (pill **reduces** the rate of the problem by the amount shown)

% rate (per 100 women) per year

Reduces heavy periods

Less benign breast disease

Eases period pains

Reduces anaemia

Lessens pre-menstrual tension

Improves acne

Less chance of ovarian cysts

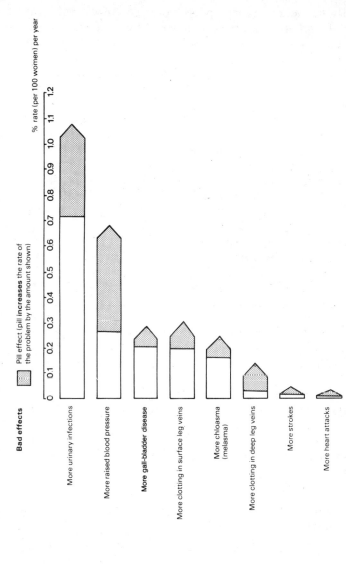

Bad effects

[shaded box] Pill effect (pill **increases** the rate of the problem by the amount shown)

% rate (per 100 women) per year

More urinary infections

More raised blood pressure

More gall-bladder disease

More clotting in surface leg veins

More chloasma (melasma)

More clotting in deep leg veins

More strokes

More heart attacks

Fig. 16 The effect of the pill on the rate of occurrence of some selected conditions (RCGP Study)

Note: All rates shown are the rates of attendance at the doctor's surgery and/or hospital admission for each condition.

The pill in perspective 161

similarly be wondering why people ever go anywhere by car? Yet all the different injuries due to cars added together are still uncommon enough to make it worth while for most people to use cars. Similarly, all the serious injuries which have been linked with the pill added together are uncommon. Indeed it would be a safe bet that most readers of this book will not know personally any family affected by a tragedy linked with the pill—whereas they probably know more than one resulting from a road accident. In spite of years of involvement with family planning, I am not aware of a case of a heart attack or stroke occurring in any woman to whom I had personally prescribed the pill (though I have been asked to look after one or two who were prescribed the pill elsewhere, after such an event).

By emphasizing the rarity of all the dangerous complications of oral contraception, the idea is to put things in perspective for the majority of actual or prospective pill-users. It is not by any means to belittle or shrug away the seriousness of the events if they do occur. Complications may be statistically rare but they are 100 per cent to the person actually affected.

Such cases would make me renew my efforts to promote the most careful possible use of the pill, as described in this book. (See particularly pages 184–5.) But they would not make me abandon the pill as an option, any more than sensible and sympathetic people after witnessing a tragic road accident would refuse ever again to travel by car. What they would do is everything in their power to help those involved, and they might then resolve to drive carefully in future, and to promote road safety.

You cannot lead your life without some risks, and when it comes to things like family planning, doing nothing can be risky too!

Why—in spite of all its known and potential unknown health risks—might I choose to use the pill?

1. *The pill is as effective as any method currently available, short of sterilization. It is highly acceptable and unrelated to intercourse. It is almost 100 per cent reversible.* (Injectables like Depo-Provera are similar, see page 255.)

2. *The pill has beneficial effects.* These are too often forgotten. They are listed in Table 7 (pages 158–9). The improvement in the symptoms of their cycle is something that is appreciated by nearly all pill-users. There are also long-term benefits such as the lowered risk of cancer of the ovary and endometrium. These are probably connected with suppressing the so-called 'normal' menstrual cycle (pages 49–50). Although some benefits are not yet proven, it is worth noting that the effect of bias, discussed on page 147, tends to hide or *underestimate* any good effects of the pill.

3. *Several times a rare event is still a rare event.* Fortunately, the serious conditions whose rate is increased by the pill, like heart attacks and strokes, are extremely rare in women of child-bearing years. So even if their rate is increased, that still makes them very rare events. Suppose the pill increases the rate of something by a huge amount, like a factor of 10. If the annual rate in non-users were 1 in 100,000, this would mean 10 cases in pill-users (i.e. 9 extra). But if the non-user rate were 10 in 100,000 there would be 100 cases per year in pill-users. The same relative risk factor of 10 means 90 extra cases in the second example but only 9 extra cases in the first. The extra cases are the so-called *attributable or excess* risk, and better convey the real importance of the pill effect. It is because the diseases are so rare making the excess risk so low for young ages that the relative risks, mostly around 2–6 for the various circulatory diseases, can be accepted. Turn back to Figure 1 (page 6) for a moment. Even for smokers under 35, for example, the excess risk for users of the old medium-to-high-oestrogen pills, for instance, is only 10 per 100,000. However, over the age of 45 it rises (not shown in the figure) to 179 per 100,000 per year.

A small extra point which is perhaps worth mentioning is that all the research that has been done on the pill has failed to show up any condition which is new to science. It was always possible that the artificial hormones of the pill might cause some completely new disease. In fact, however, all the problems that are blamed on the pill happen also to women who have never had an artificial hormone in their lives, and as far as diseases of the circulation are concerned—which are surely among the most serious alleged risks—to men too. The average man is up to three times more at risk of circulatory disease, just because of his sex, than the average woman before her menopause. So if your partner of the same age is not scared about just being a man, perhaps you (especially if free of risk factors) can be relaxed about being a pill-using woman!

4. RISK ESTIMATES ARE AVERAGES, AND DO NOT NECESSARILY APPLY TO SUB-GROUPS. To understand this point, please look back to page 98 and see how there, in the discussion on heart disease, I showed how the various estimated risks multiplied with each other and with the pill. But the opposite is also true: anyone without risk factors must have a much lower risk than average.

Perhaps an analogy may help to make this clearer. Insurance companies always require a high premium from students when they try to insure their cars; yet some of those students are very much safer drivers than the average (and may prove the fact in due course by having no accidents at all in the next 20 years). They always were safer drivers, but the risk estimates by the insurers had to be based on all kinds of students, including those who are irresponsible, who drive under the influence of alcohol, and so on. *To some considerable extent—not altogether—those for whom pill-use is especially risky can now be identified.* The next chapter is partly about how this can be done. One way of putting it is: 'The pill is reasonably safe, but some women are dangerous.' As a result of better prescribing, the 'dangerous' women either should not now be using the method or should be better monitored: and *the pill probably always was a lot less risky for the remainder (the safer women) than the overall estimates would suggest.* In fact (page 105) the heart attack risk cannot any longer be detected now except in 'the dangerous women' (chiefly smokers).

5. *The risk estimates were based on research on higher-dose pills than are now in general use.* Pills which are low in dose of oestrogen and in dose or body impact (pages 154–6) of progestogen seem, on all the new evidence becoming available, to be even safer.

However, even following all the known guidelines for increasing the safety of pill-prescribing, including careful aftercare with blood pressure checks, trouble can still strike out of a clear blue sky. Risks can be lowered, but they can never be entirely eliminated.

6. *Pregnancy is fairly risky: the pill is very effective against pregnancy: so the risks of the pill may not be so worrying when the avoidance of pregnancy is taken into consideration.* In the past, this point has sometimes been made too strongly, and various graphs and diagrams produced which suggest that non-use of the pill is more dangerous than it is. But the main point still stands, and that is that when considering methods which are not so reliable against pregnancy as the pill, we have to add together two things: (a) the risk (if any) of the method itself and (b) the risk of the pregnancies which will occur in a proportion of women due to failure of that method. No guarantee of safety can be given to any sexually active woman, whatever method of family planning she uses, or if she uses no method at all and keeps becoming pregnant. Pregnancy itself, whether its outcome is a baby or an abortion or a miscarriage, still carries some risks even in countries like Britain or America, and far more in many less developed countries (Figure 1, page 6). One way or another (and most unfairly), for women sex is dangerous.

In fact, in the real-life situations of the RCGP, Oxford/FPA, and Walnut Creek Studies the death rate due to pregnancy in the non-pill-users was extremely small. This shows that on average the women concerned, or their partners, were reasonably careful using alternative methods of family planning and they had good medical care during their pregnancies. Neither of these facts is necessarily true for other women whose circumstances or behaviour are different. The sheath, for example, can have absolutely no health risk due to the method, and used consistently its effectiveness can approach that of the IUD. Nevertheless, everyone knows that unplanned pregnancies are more frequent among users of that method, partly because the rubber of which the sheath is made may fail, but much more commonly because the user fails to use it properly or regularly. The main conclusion is that *the risk of death, whether from the method or from pregnancy if the method fails, of all the recommended methods of birth control is low, and below the risk of child-bearing* if no method is used: except for older pill-users, particularly if they smoke. This is even more true wherever medical care for pregnant women is poor, and wherever, as tragically happens in many countries, dangerous illegal or back-street abortion is widely practised. Even in countries like Britain, young women are probably exposed to less danger, particularly if they do not smoke, in any given year if they take the pill than they would be if they were to have a baby.

Yet few who want a baby are put off by these known medical risks of doing that—nor should they be. So if you are young your decision about the pill can be based more on other points, such as convenience and the fact that it almost eliminates the fear of an unwanted pregnancy.

7. *Even the highest estimates of risk due to the pill are of the same order as many other risks many of us take every day.* Most of us are extremely vague and uninformed about the relative risks of daily activities. Smoking is a good example: accepted as 'normal' yet truly lethal (page 107).

Many people accept dangers similar to or much greater than those of the pill in their occupations, spare-time activities, or hobbies. Table 8 gives some intriguing estimates derived from the *British Medical Journal*. A one in a million chance of death

Table 8 How to have a (very low) 1 in 1 million risk of dying

Activity	Distance (km)	Time required
Travel by air at 1000 km/hour (c. 600 mph)	1100	1.1 hours
By car at 100 km/hour (c. 60 mph)	100	1 hour
By motorbike at 100 km/hour (c. 60 mph)	1	< 1 minute
Rock climbing	—	1.5 minutes
Stay alive if over 65	—	5 minutes
Smoke 2 cigarettes (if a 20-a-day smoker)	—	1–2 hours
Take old-type pill (50 mcg oestrogen)	—	1 month

Source: Adapted from 'Minerva', *British Medical Journal*, 1988.

is very small. But the time to reach it can be very short (for example if you are over 65). The longest time in the Table is for young non-smoking healthy pill-takers—and that was before we had the modern, even safer pills! Can you think of anything you could do which is completely safe? How about eating? In the USA approximately 3,000 people die each year from accidentally inhaling food, usually a piece of steak . . . One would think that keeping household pets is a safe enough hobby—yet the Brompton Hospital in London has recorded at least three deaths from allergy to hamsters. See Figure 1 for some more examples (page 6).

And what about unknown risks? If you stop to think about it, which most of us do not, there are many chemicals to which we are exposed every day which have never been studied as intensively as the pill. To take a simple example, how do we know that drinking coffee is a safe habit? Until someone does something like the RCGP Study of the pill, which would mean taking 23,000 regular coffee-drinkers, and 23,000 comparable people who never touch the stuff, and then following up all 46,000 for 10 years, keeping records of every death or attack of illness in the two groups, we shall never really know. There are other unknown risks which could be a lot higher: for instance, those due to pollution. Tens of thousands of powerful chemicals are released by industry into our environment, into the water we drink and the air we breathe, and also into our food. The dose of each may be small, but *nobody knows just how much or little effect they could have on our health, either alone or in combination*. There are other chemicals to which people expose themselves voluntarily: for instance, some hair dyes have been suspected of very rarely causing cancer. Again though, no one knows how rarely. And how about the chemicals that are added to much of the food we buy? These are sometimes thought to be essential as preservatives but often they are just for colouring, such as one called Brown FK which is used solely to make kippers and ginger-nut biscuits nice and brown. Brown FK is something which could increase the rate of all kinds of diseases, and could be at least as dangerous—or as safe—as the pill. The point is we just do not know. Taking risks is quite simply part of life: or as the car-sticker puts it, 'Living is hazardous to your health.'

Please do not get me wrong: I am not arguing that two wrongs make a right, or rather that hundreds of wrongs make a right. Obviously there is no room for complacency about the risks of the pill. They should be reduced to the absolute minimum in the way that is described in the next chapter—and in the long run we hope the pill will be phased out and replaced by an entirely risk-free method (see Chapter 9). But right now the risks of the pill compare well with the known, let alone the unknown, risks to which we are all inevitably exposed. After considering its advantages and convenience, given the methods now available, the balance sheet of risks and benefits comes out favourable to the pill for many women (in their own opinion).

The effect of the mass media on people's thinking about the pill

The strange thing as I have said is that often even with known serious risks, like smoking cigarettes, so many people are quite illogically not at all bothered: and yet they are terrified by other dangers which are definitely not as great. Unbalanced press and TV publicity is often to blame. When did you last see a major article in a popular newspaper itemizing the risks of cigarettes, including interviews with the sufferers from smoking-related diseases like cancer of the lung, or with their relatives? Yet there have been numerous such articles about the pill, which quite fail to put its risks in perspective, in comparison to the risks of life generally, and especially the risks and problems of unwanted pregnancy.

It is well known that good news is not 'news'. For example, one of the good effects of the pill is the definite reduction in the chance of getting cancer of the ovary. When this was first convincingly shown the silence of the media was deafening! By contrast the FPA switchboards were jammed during the 'pill scares' about thrombosis in veins in December 1969, about heart attacks or other arterial diseases in 1977, and about breast cancer in 1983 and again in 1989. Treatment of these stories by some newspapers was so alarmist that a large number of users all over the world were frightened into stopping the pill altogether, often half-way through a packet and without taking alternative precautions. In Britain alone it is estimated that, in 1970 for example, about 20,000 babies were born as a result, not to mention the pregnancies which were terminated (abortions). In each year of panic many of those who gave up the pill were the 'wrong' people, such as healthy and thin, active, non-smoking women. The pill could have been a godsend if their confidence in it had not been shattered. Presented later with a more complete picture of the risks and other problems of the alternatives to pill-use—or sometimes learning the hard way by having to have an abortion—some of these women made the voluntary and informed choice to go back on the combined pill.

Let me make four final points. First, *coincidences do happen.* Becoming ill sometimes is part of being human. Some people are inclined to blame on the pill every illness or symptom which occurs, in a past or present user. But they fail to see the logical implication which is that never-users must never get ill at all and presumably would live for ever!

Secondly, the risk of death or serious illness; though perhaps the major concern, it is certainly not the only factor to be considered when deciding between methods of family planning. As just one example, it has been shown by several experts that one of the very safest ways of birth control from the point of view just of avoiding death is to use a simple method of family planning like a spermicide—not usually recommended for use alone—and then, whenever a pregnancy occurs, to have a legal abortion. The facts are quite correct: there is no death rate using the simple method, and the death rate from the several abortions that would be necessary if this policy were followed would also be very low. Many readers of this book may be disturbed if not horrified by this suggestion; other might feel less strongly but would agree that this is simply not the right way to go about things. Abortion is not family planning, though it is a fact that the difference between the two is becoming increasingly difficult to define (see page 235). Many, perhaps most, women would feel very uneasy if this approach were seriously recommended to them. That is not to say that some would not feel that an abortion was right in certain particular circumstances: it is the planning to have abortions regularly that would seem so wrong to many. I use this example chiefly to show that in the real world risks are not necessarily the most important factors which people consider when deciding what they themselves are going to do.

Thirdly, if one day a new contraceptive medicine which affects the whole system like the pill is devised, it will be worth considering the saying 'better the devil you know than the devil you don't'. In other words, we now know a lot about the pill which will inevitably take a long time to emerge during use of a new drug. It may perhaps be said of such a new drug that it is believed to have no unwanted effects on the circulation or on breast cancer. That could be true, but then it might eventually prove to have more serious effects elsewhere in the body. 'Newer' is not necessarily 'better'.

Finally, in spite of what I have just said, as we saw earlier there are still many gaps in our knowledge about the pill itself. There are two ways of reacting to absent facts about the use of any drug, or of the pill. One person may say, *'there is not enough evidence of safety'*, another may say, *'there is no evidence of danger'*. A good example of what I mean can be found on page 222 of this book. A microscopic amount of progestogen gets into the breast milk if a woman is on the progestogen-only pill while breast-feeding. There is so far nothing to suggest that this could harm the baby in any way: but, of course, it might. I myself would say, 'there is no evidence that this harms the baby' and therefore I do prescribe this kind of pill at the request of a breast-feeding mother, after discussing the arguments with her. But others might react by saying 'there is no proof that this is entirely harmless to the baby': and this is an equally true statement, just the other way round. It is a bit like the difference between saying that a bottle is 'half full' and 'half empty'.

The point is that we are all having to decide on the basis of the *same* present and absent facts. At the end of the day, it is a question of judgement. There are bound to be honest differences of opinion about how pills should be used—at least until the facts become absolutely unarguable, which is a rare event in the whole of medicine.

7

Who for the pill, and which pill for you?

Who should never take the pill?

We now know much better than before which women should never take the pill. If these are identified and advised to use other methods, then the remainder can use the pill with added confidence.

Whether the method is really to be forbidden in particular circumstances, or could perhaps be used with special care, is something about which experts frequently disagree. Opinions also change as more research is done. My own advice is different today from that in earlier editions. I think most doctors would agree with me in 1991 that another method should always be used if anyone comes into one of the following categories. They are often called *absolute contra-indications*.

1. Past or present serious disease affecting the circulation

(a) *Past history of any form of thrombosis* in any artery or vein anywhere in the body (see Chapter 4). The pill should be avoided whether the clotting occurred while previously taking the pill, whether in a situation which makes clotting more likely such as pregnancy or being confined to bed after an operation, or completely unexpectedly. All these troubles are rare, but the least uncommon would be clotting in one of the leg veins (pages 94–5).

(b) *Any past history of brain trouble diagnosed as a stroke* (pages 99–100), whether thought to be due to blood clotting or to bleeding in the brain.

(c) *Extremely severe, so-called 'crescendo' migraine*; any

migraine bad enough to be *treated with an ergotamine-containing drug* (page 111); or *migraine of the focal type*. Focal migraine shows itself by short-lived attacks of strange and very worrying symptoms (see page 100). There is a risk that these could lead to an actual stroke in a woman on the pill. So any woman with migraine of this most unusual kind should either never go on the pill, or discontinue if she is already on it when the attack happens.

The same applies if such symptoms were ever to occur without a headache at all—this is thought to happen if there is a temporary interruption to the blood supply (ischaemia) of the brain; such attacks are labelled *transient ischaemic attacks*.

(d) *An illness or condition which makes thrombosis more likely e.g. 'large dose' of a risk factor for disease of the circulation* (see page 97). What matters is how bad the risk factor is, and again, I think, most experts would agree that the following should avoid the pill:

- A woman who has a known problem of *high or abnormal blood fats*. She may be on a special diet and possibly drug treatment for it already, since it often runs in families. Other causes include some long-term kidney and bowel diseases. See pages 87, 90, 97 and 178.

- *A woman with severe diabetes, who already has signs of damage to the arteries, nerves, or kidneys or changes affecting the eye*.

- A woman with *high blood pressure*, even when not on the pill. If there is a past history of blood pressure going up very significantly on the pill, and returning to normal when it was stopped, this also means that the combined pill should be avoided in future. Repeated readings at or above 160 mm for the systolic or 95 mm for the diastolic pressures—explained on page 103—would in my view be too high both for starting and for continuing with the pill.

- *A very heavy cigarette smoker (40 or more cigarettes a day)*. Under age 30, short-term use of a brand with one of the 'lipid-friendly' progestogens (pages 155–6) might just be permissible.

- *A grossly obese woman* (say weighing over 50 per cent more than the correct weight for her height).

The above examples are where the single risk factor is strong enough on its own. More commonly, the decision to avoid the pill is based on:

- *Combinations of risk factors.* If two or more of the factors just mentioned apply, then the woman should avoid the pill completely, even though on their own they would not be bad enough for this to be recommended. For instance, any diabetic on treatment who is also a long-term smoker of 15 cigarettes or more should, in my view, avoid the method. You can easily work out other combinations which mean the same thing.

- *Angina.* This means heart pain, of a type which is usually described as a constricting feeling around the chest, and perhaps going up the neck or down the arms, which is brought on by exercise. If this diagnosis has been given to such a pain, it means that the heart muscle is being temporarily supplied with too little blood. This happens because the coronary (heart) arteries are already affected by atherosclerosis, i.e. hardening of the arteries. So to reduce the chances of an actual coronary thrombosis, which would block the arteries altogether, the pill is certainly best avoided if any woman has been told she has angina.

* - *Some rarities.* This means other types of *heart disease*, including most varieties affecting the heart valves; *pulmonary hypertension* (high blood pressure in the circulation through the lungs); a type of irregular heartbeat called *atrial fibrillation*; known *abnormalities of blood clotting factors*; and after *surgical removal of the spleen* if the number of platelets (page 93) is above the normal range.

* The pill should be avoided altogether in those of the rare so-called *connective tissue diseases*, such as SLE and polyarteritis nodosa, and in some *blood diseases* —leukaemia, polycythaemia—in which there is already an increased likelihood of thrombosis.

The combined pill should also normally be avoided or stopped in three life circumstances in which the risk of thrombosis is increased—particularly in veins of the legs (pages 94–5):

- *Living above a height of 4,000 metres.* This can raise blood viscosity and make clotting more likely. It is probably not necessary to stop the pill if you are young and fit and plan to trek in the Himalayas, since the vigorous exercise would be protective. But it would be important if you were to be sedentary at high altitude. See also page 278 re long-haul plane journeys.

- *Immobilization in bed, such as after an accident.* Disabled women who are confined to a wheelchair may, however, be permitted to take an ultra-low-dose combined pill provided they are not overweight, and with special medical supervision.

- *For four weeks before and at least two weeks after you are fully mobile following any planned major operation or any surgery to the legs (especially orthopaedic surgery).* Varicose vein treatments, whether by injections or surgery, also mean stop the pill (page 96). The main thing for you to check with the surgeon is if the complication of leg thrombosis is particularly linked with the planned operation or treatment. *Emergency* operations can of course still be done, but it is vital to inform the doctor on your admission that you are taking the pill in case blood thinning with a drug called heparin is required. Sterilization by laparoscopy (page 236) does not cause thrombosis so the combined pill need not be stopped beforehand.

As the progestogen-only pill (page 217) and Depo-Provera (page 255) do not contain oestrogen and are not thought to affect clotting factors to any important extent, most doctors agree that they can be continued up to and after major as well as minor operations. Indeed either could be ideal to tide you over the whole time on the waiting list, in hospital, and until you restart the ordinary pill. This would normally be on the first day of your next period which is at least two weeks after you are able to walk around. But with the Depo-Provera the pill could be started any time, even without waiting for the injection's 12 weeks of effectiveness to come to an end, if you prefer.

2. Present disease of the liver—whether or not connected with the pill

If are still suffering from the effects of damage to your liver after any kind of liver illness such as jaundice (commonly caused by *infectious hepatitis*), then the pill like alcohol should be avoided—normally for three months after the relevant blood tests have become normal. Further tests of liver function may be advised after a month or so of pill-taking.

- The type of *jaundice of pregnancy* described on page 117 is so likely to recur on the pill that it would be sensible to avoid it.
* - The disease *cirrhosis* of the liver, rare conditions of the liver and skin known as the *porphyrias*, and a couple of *exotic disorders affecting the excretion of bile*, e.g. *Rotor syndrome, all contra-indicate the pill.*
* - A history of one of the very rare *tumours of the liver* (page 145) means another method for the future.
- Finally, *gallstones* treated medically in the past could recur within the bile duct system, so it would normally be best to avoid the pill in future. See page 117. The pill should be usable if the treatment was by removal of the gall-bladder, but check this with your surgeon.

*3. Past history of actual cancer of any type which might be aggravated by the hormones of the pill

The reason is that the hormones of the pill *might* make the cancer more difficult to cure. The rule particularly applies to those very few women of child-bearing years who have had cancer of the breast. The treatment of most gynaecological cancers (cervix, endometrium, or ovary) involves removing the uterus (hysterectomy), so there is then no need to use the pill for family planning. Otherwise it is best if any woman who has had cancer of any type takes the advice of the specialist looking after her, and avoids the pill until she is given the 'all clear'. See also page 183 below.

4. Recent abnormal bleeding, other than at period times, from the uterus: until its cause has been found

The reason for avoiding the pill here is that any vaginal bleeding which is not clearly connected with periods—especially if it happens after intercourse—must be diagnosed as quickly as possible. This is to rule out disease of the uterus, commonly non-malignant growths called polyps, but very, very rarely cancer. As irregular bleeding of the type known as 'break-through' bleeding can occur on the pill, if this rule were not followed there is a risk that the diagnosis would be delayed, because the bleeding might be thought to be a side-effect of the pill. However, once the gynaecologist has definitely ruled out a serious cause for the abnormal bleeding, he will almost certainly then be happy for you to take the pill.

5. Actual or possible pregnancy

Here the reason for avoiding the pill until pregnancy has been ruled out is that there is an unproven risk, which if it exists must be very, very small, that pill-taking during pregnancy might damage the baby (see pages 129–30).

6. Past history of any serious condition occurring or worsening in a previous pregnancy, and/or known to be affected by sex hormones

This is because, as I have said, the pill in some ways mimics pregnancy. *Jaundice of pregnancy* (page 117), the troublesome skin rash called *herpes gestationis* (page 135), and *chorea* (page 113) are three examples mentioned earlier. Deterioration of the inherited form of deafness called *otosclerosis* has been reported in pregnancy, so again the pill is usually avoided; though in fact no increase in the number of patients with this trouble was shown among pill-takers in the RCGP Study.

*7. Recent trophoblastic disease

This was explained on page 145. Because of the risk of a rare cancer following it, *in this country* it is still recommended that oral contraception should be avoided, but only until the special follow-up tests of hCG hormone levels are completely normal. After that, provided your gynaecologist agrees, the pill can be used in the normal way.

8. Important condition occurring on the pill in the past and considered to be due to it

High blood pressure which definitely seems in a particular case to be related to taking the pill has already been mentioned above; another example would be *bad migraine* occurring on the pill in a woman who never used to have the problem. This category also includes other conditions which can be found in Chapter 5, if your doctor feels that the pill is very likely to blame: for example, the severe skin rash *erythema multiforme*, which may be due to an allergy to one of the hormones contained in the pill.

9. Unconvinced that the pill is right for you

If you or your partner cannot feel confident about using the pill, after discussing things with your doctor, or reading a book like this, then obviously you should avoid it. A doctor may perhaps insist that there is no medical reason why you should not take it, but you should always have the final word.

Notice, by the way, that several of the above reasons for avoiding the pill are not necessarily permanent.

Who should be very cautious about taking the pill and then only with special medical supervision? (See pages 184–5 for what is meant by 'special supervision')

This means women with *relative contra-indications:* risk factors which do not necessarily mean that the pill should be avoided altogether, but which do require careful consideration *relative* to the other risks—including those of pregnancy—that are faced by that woman, and the acceptability of alternatives to the pill.

For example, diabetes in a young woman increases the risk of disease of the circulation, as does the pill (page 97); but it also increases the risks of pregnancy and delivery above the average. So if no other acceptable method can be found the pill could still be a reasonable choice for short-term use after discussion and with careful medical supervision.

These relative contra-indications are mostly obvious after reading Chapters 4 and 5. The important ones are listed here: if more than one applies, particularly of the first seven below, then the pressure to move to another method rather than the pill increases.

1. A family history of disease of the circulation

This means a history of thrombosis—such as coronary thrombosis or deep-vein thrombosis in the legs—or of stroke, occurring in a near-relative *at a young age*: say under 45. Such diseases in young member(s) of your family may mean artery trouble and, unless you live where the tests are not available, your doctor will arrange for measurements of clotting factors and blood fats (page 97). Should abnormal levels be found, then you will be told to avoid the *combined* pill (see pages 172, 220). If not, and in cases where the family history is not so strong, the pill may be used with special supervision.

The doctor should also be told if there is a tendency in your family to raised blood pressure.

2. Diabetes—but also see page 172

Diseases of the circulation are already more likely in diabetics, so in my view it is preferable to avoid any extra risk in the same direction. In practice, however, some young diabetics who are free of any signs of complications of the disease (page 172) do use the pill, because they need maximum protection against pregnancy. There may be no satisfactory alternative. If so they occasionally need to increase their insulin dose and they should naturally be seen at frequent intervals by a doctor. It is even more crazy for diabetics to smoke than it is for other people: and if they do they certainly should not use the pill. Otherwise they should be on the lowest possible dose of pill, ideally using a new lipid-friendly progestogen (page 155) or even better the POP (page 221), and for as short a time as possible. They will probably be encouraged to have their babies as young as their circumstances allow. Then they will most likely be advised to transfer to another method or perhaps be sterilized as soon as they complete their family.

Women with a strong family history of diabetes, or who are overweight, or who had the very mild blood test changes of diabetes in pregnancy, or who gave birth to a baby weighing more than 4.5 kg, all need to be carefully observed on the pill. For *some* of these, it may be right to have the test mentioned on page 88 (the Glucose Tolerance Test) before and perhaps a couple of months after going on the combined pill. But *all* should especially beware of putting on too much weight . . .

3. High blood pressure—see also page 172

Everything really depends on how bad the blood pressure is, how young the woman is, whether there are any other risk factors present, and whether any alternative methods of family planning are acceptable. Readings *around* 140 systolic/90 diastolic (page 102) will normally indicate just frequent check-ups. If you have higher levels your doctor may advise you to abandon the combined pill; and this would certainly be necessary if the values were above 160/95. You might then try the progestogen-only type (Chapter 8). It is important to remember that a rise in blood pressure may sometimes be an *early warning sign* (see page 102). So even a small rise can be important if there are other risk factors already—e.g. in a smoker.

A past history of *raised blood pressure during pregnancy* ('toxaemia') has recently (1989) been shown by the RCGP researchers to increase the risk of heart attacks enormously, especially in smokers. However the extra risk due to pill-taking in smokers (they could not show any problem at all in non-smokers) did not seem to be different with that pregnancy history. So as with a past history of *kidney disease*, the pill is an option—but with caution, strong advice to cut down/out smoking, and more frequent checks of the blood pressure during early months of use.

*4. Sickle cell anaemia

This is a type of anaemia which affects only black people. There are two forms of the condition and the milder one, which is pretty common, called sickle cell *trait*, definitely poses no problem for pill-taking. But experts disagree about whether it must be avoided by patients with the rare sickle cell *anaemia*.

They have attacks (so-called crises) from time to time, during which damaged red blood cells block up tiny arteries in the body. Theoretically these attacks might be worsened by oestrogen, promoting thrombosis and thus turning temporary blockages of the microcirculation into more permanent ones. Other evidence suggests that the progestogen of the pill might have favourable effects.

Since pregnancy is particularly dangerous in this condition, many experts now allow or even prefer a low-dose pill to be used—after full discussion. This makes it only a relative contra-indication. In this country it remains more usual to prescribe either the POP (Chapter 8) or a quite different method. A particularly good choice might be Depo-Provera (page 255). Research reported in 1982 showed this injectable contraceptive can be positively beneficial to women with sickle cell anaemia, by reducing the frequency of their painful crises.

5. Cigarette-smoking; Age; Duration of use

This was all discussed fully on pages 149–52. The 'bottom line' was that *smokers* must stop the ordinary combined pill at 35 and should not use it for more than 15 years maximum. *Non-smokers* now have no absolute age or duration limits, if they choose (because of the pill's benefits) voluntarily to take the small increasing risk of circulatory diseases which does occur with increasing age up to the menopause.

6. Migraine

The problematic migraines were fully discussed on pages 101, 112. But even migraines without special 'focal' symptoms are a reason for some caution. Sufferers need to be taught the symptoms to look out for which would mean taking prompt advice (pages 75, 101). And remember the usefulness of *tricycling* if the bad headaches are nearly always during the pill-free gap between active tablets (page 52).

7. Excessive weight (page 98); Marked varicose veins (pages 95–6)

These were discussed earlier. Both tend to be associated with an increased risk of thrombosis, but probably indirectly. Both can also become more problematic in pill-takers. Overweight is of course something about which you can, in theory, do something yourself.

For women in all the above categories a pill which is particularly low in oestrogen and combined with a new 'lipid-friendly' progestogen is preferable, as explained on pages 155–6. Now I come on to some reasons for extra caution which are not to do with diseases of the circulation.

8. Scanty or very irregular periods or their absence (amenorrhoea)

Following use of the pill, lack of egg-release and therefore of periods for six months to a year or longer does occur in a very few women (see page 77). Some of these may require special treatment in order to achieve a pregnancy, but the success rate in good centres now approaches 100 per cent. Such women should not worry that taking the pill has caused their problem and wrecked their chances of having a baby.

It is illogical for the combined pill to be used simply to 'regularize' infrequent, irregular periods. After all, 'pill periods' are entirely artificial (see page 47). However, women currently seeing no periods or less than four periods a year and not yet wanting a baby should be referred for full investigation, and then may well be allowed the pill as an *option*. Indeed, sometimes the tests demonstrate that the pill would be positively beneficial!

If the doctor finds no special reason to prescribe oestrogen or progestogen (in the pill, as therapy), what alternative contraception might be used? The best, if acceptable, would be barriers such as the sheath or the cap, or even (so long as the amenorrhoea which means very reduced fertility continues) just the sponge (page 250). The IUD would be a very poor choice as it is linked with a risk of blocked tubes—a much less treatable cause of reduced fertility (see pages 252, 256–7).

In teenagers, starting the pill should always be delayed until periods have appeared. Otherwise there are no proven *medical* risks at this age, though there is the concern about breast cancer (page 139). See also pages 23–31, 82, 133.

*9. Present disorder of the pituitary gland

This is a rare reason for going on the pill, and the woman concerned should already be seeing a specialist. A woman with this problem may be told she is infertile. But if there are high blood levels of the hormone prolactin (page 131), pregnancy is very possible especially when treatment begins. Present advice is to use the pill in some cases but only under the supervision of a specialist.

10. Fluid retention

Too much fluid in the body can be risky for a few people who have certain types of *heart and kidney disease*. The pill tends to cause retention of some fluid (page 92) so special care is needed.

11. Severe depression (see page 108)

A history of really bad depression which required treatment for a long time with drugs for 'nerves' means caution. But unplanned pregnancy is depressing; and the Oxford/FPA study showed (in 1985) no link at all between the pill and severe depression or other 'serious' psychiatric illness.

12. The use of interfering drugs—especially treatments for tuberculosis and epilepsy (see page 71, also 196–7)

Page 70 lists those drugs which may cause problems. The main thing is to make sure that the doctor who prescribes you the pill knows what, if any, other drugs you take; and if you are about to start any new treatment, to remind the doctor that you are a pill-taker. As explained on page 71, there is no problem if you have acne and have already taken tetracycline for more than four weeks. But if the interfering treatment is an 'enzyme inducer' (page 71) to be used long term, as in epilepsy, and alternative methods do not suit you, special pill-taking advice applies. The tricycle regimen (page 52) is now recommended, for the reasons explained on pages 59–64, with a pill-free break of only five days between each 'run' of three packets. And (unusually) it is best for you to use one of the 50 mcg pills from Table 10 (page 188) rather than the generally preferred ultra-low-dose pills of Table 9. This is because of the need to overcome the effect of the interference by the other drug which may be causing the pill to be less effective.

It is also very important for you to go back promptly to your clinic or family doctor if you ever get 'breakthrough' bleeding or fail to get a 'period'. In that event (assuming the pill has not failed) you may rarely even have to be recommended to take two pills a day to overcome completely the weakening effect of the interfering drug.

13. Previous failure of the pill (pregnancy while taking it)

The answer especially if you keep forgetting tablets may be another method altogether, such as the injection (page 255) or an IUD. But your very ability to get pregnant by missing an occasional pill (lots of people do and get away with it) may mean you are someone whose metabolism gets rid of the pill hormones from your body extra rapidly. So to improve your 'margin for error' I now recommend tricycling the pill (pages 52–3), which means having fewer of the 'contraceptively dangerous' pill-free breaks from pill-taking. This is explained on pages 59–64. You may also need to take a stronger pill and must try extra hard to remember it too, of course!

*14. Should the pill be used by people who already have other chronic (long-term) diseases?

It all depends. There is obviously no space to consider them all here, but if you look in the Index you will find that a number, such as diabetes and Crohn's disease (page 116), have already been discussed. Some women who have diseases which lead to very heavy periods, such as those on artificial kidney treatment —or who have difficulty because of disablement in coping with naturally rather heavy periods—positively benefit from the light ones that the pill gives. If women with the allergic and auto-immune disorders considered on page 137 go on the pill, the result is often unpredictable, so close medical supervision is essential. Melanoma (page 145), most cancers, Hodgkin's disease, multiple sclerosis, myasthenia gravis, and sarcoidosis are examples of illnesses which are now believed to be neither worsened nor improved by the pill. But more research is needed, into these and others too numerous to mention.

The main rules are:

(a) discuss the whole matter with your doctor, as usual balancing known and potential unknown risks of the pill *in your situation* against those of pregnancy and the pros and cons of alternative methods;

(b) be sure that you are *carefully followed up* by a doctor or specialist who knows the full story.

15. Abnormal cervical smears under observation or treated (see page 142)

The pill may continue to be used at the woman's choice during investigation for an abnormality in a cervical smear test, or following successful treatment whether by the laser or a cone biopsy (removal of the affected skin under anaesthetic), or the equivalent. All experts are agreed that *attending without fail for the follow-up smears as instructed* (usually annually) is the first priority. This gives such safe monitoring of the situation that if a woman really wants to continue taking the pill, she may do so. Or she might decide after full discussion to use a barrier in future (as well, or instead): this would have the advantage of protecting the cervix from the cause of the abnormal cells (page 28). The choice is up to her. She would be mad to continue smoking (page 143) . . .

16. Breast cancer in close relative(s); or benign breast disease (risk factors)

To play safe, while awaiting more research, relatively short-term use is advised if the pill is used. See pages 138–40, 141, 142.

How then can use of the pill be made safer? An ideal scheme

- First of all, *women to whom something applies from the first list above* (pages 171–7) *should use some other method*.
- *Secondly, those with relative contra-indications* (pages 177–84) *should either avoid it or use it under special*

medical supervision. This means being seen at a clinic or surgery more often than usual, being told if there is anything special to look out for so as to return earlier if necessary, and sometimes having special tests done. It also means being ready to discontinue the pill should a condition worsen, or a new risk factor or problem appear—such as raised blood pressure.

- Thirdly, *all women, especially those with risk factors, should use pills with the lowest acceptable* (see pages 200–2) *amount or body impact of both hormones—with duration of use being periodically reassessed* (page 151).

- Fourthly, *all pill-users should be seen regularly* by a trained person who can answer their questions, and check their weight and *especially their blood pressure* (page 153). Every pill-user should be able to contact the trained person at short notice should a symptom arise—whether it is an annoying or irritating one, or a worrying one such as those in the list on page 75. This would sometimes be for a change of pill or a change of method, but often for simple reassurance. Particularly important to report is the first onset of *migraine headaches* while on the pill, or any change in related symptoms (page 101). Pill-users should also practise monthly *self-examination of the breasts* (page 142) and have regular *cervical smears* (page 81).

In summary, the SAFER women (see page 164) should use the modern SAFER pills, with careful MONITORING.

What pills are available?

Table 9 lists those pills containing less than 50 mcg of oestrogen which are currently available in Britain. This category includes the first-choice pills for all women. They do provide enough hormones to be extremely effective against pregnancy. Provided they are taken regularly, they seem to be as effective for most women as the pills containing 50 mcg of oestrogen which are all shown in Table 10. However, the 'room-for-error' factor is probably less. So it is even more important that pills are not taken late or missed. Secondly, the main reason for choosing from these pills is that, as they give less total hormone dose,

*Table 9 Ultra-low-dose combined pills with less than 50 mcg of oestrogen available in the UK

Name of pill	Dose of oestrogen (ethinyloestradiol) (mcg)	Name and dose of progestogen (mcg)	Remarks
Group A			
Cilest	35	*norgestimate* 250	Available abroad, planned for UK market
Group B		*gestodene*	
Minulet			
Femodene	30	75	
Femodene ED			
Group C		*desogestrel*	
Marvelon	30	150	
Mercilon	20	150	
Group D		*levonorgestrel*	
Ovran 30	30	250	
Eugynon 30			
Ovranette	30	150	
Microgynon 30			
Trinordiol	30, 40, 30 [32.4]	50, 75, 125 [92]	Doses are for first 6 days, then 5 days, then 10 days, respectively
Logynon			
Logynon ED			

Group E

		norethisterone	
Norimin ⎫	35	1000	
Neocon 1/35 ⎬			
Binovum	35, 35 [35]	500, 1000 [833]	Doses are for first 7 days, then 14 days, respectively
TriNovum	35, 35, 35 [35]	500, 750, 1000 [750]	Each dose for 7 days
Synphase	35, 35, 35 [35]	500, 1000, 500 [714]	Doses are for 7, then 9, then 5 days, respectively
Brevinor ⎫	35	500	
Ovysmen ⎬			

Group E (cont.)   *norethisterone acetate*

Loestrin 30	30	1500
Loestrin 20	20	1000

Group E (cont.)   *ethynodiol diacetate*

Conova 30	30	2000

Notes: 1. Each group used a different progestogen All are 21-day regimens.
2. The pills which are bracketed together have icentical formulas, and the main difference is that they are marketed by different firms.
3. Within the body, all the progestogens in pills in Group E are largely converted into norethisterone.
4. *Average* daily doses of phasic pills are in square brackets.
5. 'ED' (Every Day) versions have 7 blank or dummy tablets of lactose for the no-treatment days.

Table 10 'Ordinary' low-dose combined pills—all containing 50 mcg of oestrogen—available in the UK

Name of pill	Name and dose of progestogen (mcg)	Remarks
Group D Ovran	levonorgestrel 250	
Group E Norinyl-1 Ortho-Novin 1/50 }	norethisterone 1000	Both contain mestranol —as the oestrogen— this becomes ethinyloestradiol in the body
Group E (cont.) Anovlar 21 Gynovlar 21 Norlestrin Orlest 21 Minovlar Minovlar ED }	norethisterone acetate 4000 3000 2500 1000	All removed from UK market since last edition, purely for commercial reasons
Group E (cont.) Ovulen 50	ethynodiol diacetate 1000	
Group E (cont.) Minilyn	lynestrenol 1000	

See notes 1–3 of Table 9.

they should according to present knowledge give rise to less unwanted effects—both of the dangerous and 'nuisance' type. But the Table 9 pills are not all equivalent. There are some (notably Eugynon 30/Ovran 30 and Conova 30) which have greater unwanted effects on blood fats and insulin than the others and should therefore be avoided (page 154), unless there is a special reason (such as those discussed on page 203).

Tables 9 and 10, and Figure 17—which is about to be explained—are based on those pills at present available in Britain. However, if you live elsewhere, you should still be able to follow the discussion in the rest of this chapter if you refer to the World directory of pill names (page 301). This shows the individual formulations and the brand names used all over the world, including those equivalent to the ones in the Tables and Figures. Perhaps the simplest thing would be to use a ball-point pen to change the names here to those given to the brands used in your country.

Pill ladders

Please look at Figure 17: you will find it useful to keep referring to it throughout the rest of this chapter. The pills from both Tables 9 and 10 have been brought together in this figure, and those which contain the same progestogen in each of the Groups A to E have been arranged in ladders, also labelled A to E. They are ranked one above the other like the rungs of a ladder, in approximate order of total hormone dose being given to the body. The recommended pills are below the second horizontal line, and below them—'at ground level' so to speak because so little hormone is being taken—are the progestogen-only pills.

The main message of Figure 17 is that, like all ladders, the lower down you are the less risk there is. For most women a pill below the *second* line in the figure is preferable, thus excluding the brands in the middle section (Eugynon 30/Ovran 30 and Conova 30, see above).

Within any one ladder, the ranking order is clear, as you can see by checking the doses given in Tables 9 and 10. The oestrogen mestranol in Norinyl-1 and in Ortho-Novin 1/50 ends up, after conversion in the body, mainly as the standard oestrogen of all the other pills, ethinyloestradiol.

Ladders A, B, and C are different

The three progestogens used in these modern pills are different: they appear to be more 'selective'. This means they give more of the contraceptive and bleeding cycle controlling effects women want, but less of the unwanted effects particularly on blood fats (lipids). Norgestimate (ladder A) is available in continental Europe, but had not yet reached the UK market by the beginning of 1991.

Gestodene (GSD) is so far available in only one combination, Femodene/Minulet, with a particularly good reputation for cycle control. Desogestrel (DSG) is in Marvelon and also in Mercilon which has only 20 mcg of oestrogen. That one is especially

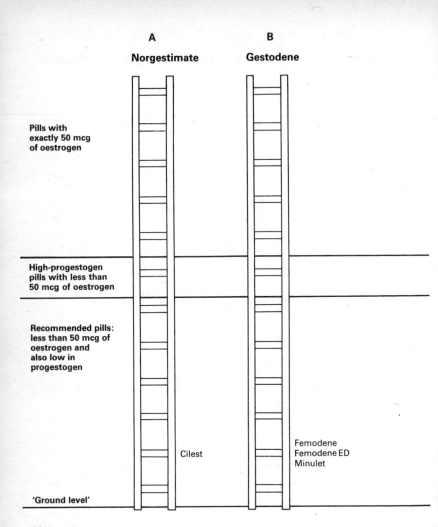

Fig. 17 Pill ladders

Notes: 1. Within each ladder the same progestogen is used.
2. The rungs are ranked as far as possible according to the total hormone dose being

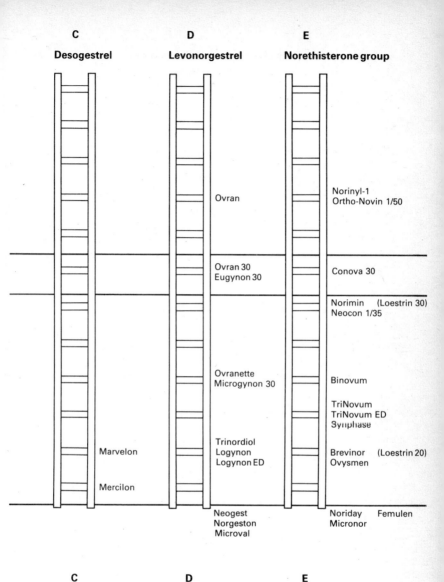

C	D	E
Desogestrel	**Levonorgestrel**	**Norethisterone group**

	Ovran	Norinyl-1 Ortho-Novin 1/50
	Ovran 30 Eugynon 30	Conova 30
		Norimin (Loestrin 30) Neocon 1/35
	Ovranette Microgynon 30	Binovum
		TriNovum TriNovum ED Synphase
Marvelon	Trinordiol Logynon Logynon ED	Brevinor (Loestrin 20) Ovysmen
Mercilon		
	Neogest Norgeston Microval	Noriday Femulen Micronor

C   D   E

given: lowest = least dose. Loestrin 20 and 30 are difficult to classify: very low/low oestrogen dose but a medium to high dose of progestogen.

3. Refer to the World directory of pill names (page 301) if living outside the UK.

Who for the pill, and which pill?   191

useful wherever there are reasons for making the oestrogen dose as low as possible—especially in overweight women and older women (page 258). Unlike Loestrin 20 (Table 9), which has a rather poor reputation, it gives reasonably good cycle control, though it is less good than Marvelon. We await a similar product using gestodene, to give women more choice, and it is a pity that so far no manufacturer has created a proper 'ladder' for the newest progestogens by giving us a 50 mcg oestrogen version for special cases (pages 182–3, and 196).

Other DSG- and GSD-containing pills are still being developed, including a progestogen-only version. But already those we have are in my opinion the first-choice types for all women with a risk factor for arterial disease (pages 97–9). Others may use them too, or alternatively any of those as near to the bottom of ladder D or E as they find acceptable (see below).

Phasic pills—triphasic or biphasic brands

Phasic pills are low-dose varieties in which the ratio of the progestogen to the oestrogen is not fixed, as normally, but is made to change at least once during each 21-day course of pills. There is a stepwise increase in the progestogen dose at each change, so that there is less in the first phase than in the second (biphasic pills), or in the second and usually the third phases (triphasic pills). See Table 9, pages 186–7, for the actual doses used.

Although like all combined pills the phasic types take away the menstrual cycle (page 47), the hormones are given in a way which does somewhat imitate the normal monthly variations. There is no evidence this is better for general health. But under the microscope a more normal-looking lining to the uterus does develop, and comes away better during each 'period' (withdrawal bleed). So although they give such a small and therefore probably safer dose of the progestogens that they use (page 155), they give a better bleeding pattern than similar fixed-dose versions would. For example, Trinordiol/Logynon is as good for this as the higher-dose and increasingly therefore less popular Ovranette/Microgynon 30.

Studies of the body chemistry of users of phasic pills have

tended to show reduced effects (sometimes no effects) on important substances such as HDL_2-cholesterol (page 154), as compared with comparable fixed-dose brands. This is chiefly because the latter have to give a higher dose to control bleeding. But the new, more selective progestogens of ladders A, B, and C can achieve similar or even better body chemistry results even in monophasic versions.

With phasic pills treatment normally *starts* on the first day of a period, with no extra precautions necessary—unless it is the Every Day type (follow the rules of the package insert). Always take the phases of pills in the correct order, as shown by the arrows.

If transferring from another pill higher up a ladder, it is best to follow the rule on page 72—i.e. immediate transfer from the last pill of the old packet to the first of the phasic pill, again with no extra precautions. Take your doctor's advice if transferring to an Every Day variety. If you transfer on the particular day during the last week of the previous pill packet which allows you to take the first *active* hormone-containing pill without there being any break between packets, no extra precautions will be required. In the case of Logynon ED this means *starting with the first (pink) Saturday tablet in the sequence, having stopped the previous brand whenever you reached the last Friday pill*—i.e. generally wasting the last few tablets in the previous packet. If, however, you follow the rules of the package insert, you will start on the first day of your withdrawal bleed after the previous packet. As this usually means taking some 'dummy' pills first, another method such as the sheath should then be used as well for the next 14 days. The reason for these extra precautions is explained on page 72.

It will obviously be easier to understand the last paragraph if you have the relevant pill packets in front of you.

Now for a summary of the main pros and cons of these pills.

Advantages of phasic pills

1. Little effect on most substances measured in the blood. But this is also true of some other ultra-low-dose brands giving a fixed dose (which may otherwise suit the woman).

2. *Almost* 100 per cent effective, like other pills, if taken regularly (but see below).

3. Good control of the bleeding pattern.

4. Logynon and Trinordiol are relatively oestrogen dominant (page 204) compared with the nearest equivalent in Figure 17.

5. Unproven: long-term benefits due to imitating the menstrual cycle(?).

Problems of phasic pills

1. Reduced margin for error if women tend to forget pills.

2. Rather easier to get confused and hence to make pill-taking errors, as there are two or three phases (or even four in ED versions!) to take in the right order. Each phase attracts a dispensing fee so they are also relatively more expensive for the NHS when issued through any chemist. What is more, unhelpfully some versions do not have the day of the week against the tablet.

3. Explaining how to use them takes a bit more of the doctor's or nurse's time.

4. Some women complain of pre-menstrual symptoms during the final phase of tablet-taking, such as breast tenderness.

5. A very few women transferring from fixed-dose pills complain of a heavier or more painful flow during periods.

6. Phasic pills are not a good choice if progestogen dominance is required (page 203).

7. They are not suitable for tricycling (pages 52–3), and even just postponing a period is more complicated than with fixed-dose pills. Page 53 describes the usual way to do this, by taking two packets in a row. With a phasic pill (except Synphase whose third phase is identical to the first)) that might well not work; the switch from the higher progestogen dose of the last phase to the low dose of the first phase tends to cause withdrawal bleeding. So there are two options (see Figure 18):

(a) *Take extra pills from the last phase of a different packet.* This will give a maximum of 10 days' postponement with Trinordiol/Logynon, for example, using the yellow tablets; or seven days using the third phase of Trinovum (which can be conveniently snapped off).

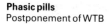

Phasic pills
Postponement of WTB

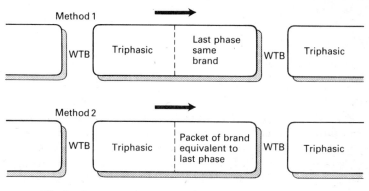

Method 1

| WTB | Triphasic | Last phase same brand | WTB | Triphasic |

Method 2

| WTB | Triphasic | Packet of brand equivalent to last phase | WTB | Triphasic |

NB - For Synphase just run on packets

Fig. 18 Two possible methods for short-term postponement of withdrawal bleeding (WTB) by women using phasic pills. The brand 'equivalent to the last phase' will be a monophasic pill with a (near-) identical formulation, e.g. Microgynon / Ovranette in the case of the triphasic levonorgestrel pills, Logynon / Trinordiol.

(b) *Interpose a packet of the next higher brand up the same ladder* in Figure 17. You should make an 'instant' switch from the phasic pill to the fixed-dose brand—i.e. no days without pill-taking till the end of a 42-tablet sequence. This should give at least six weeks free of bleeding.

Example: The very next day after her last Trinovum pill on, say, a Monday, Mrs Jones takes the first pill (marked Tuesday) from a Norimin packet. Three weeks later she takes the last Norimin on her usual finishing day, a Monday, and expects to bleed during the usual seven-day break thereafter. Then she goes back to her usual triphasic brand, taking the Tuesday pill from the first (white) section of another Trinovum packet. Contraceptive protection will continue uninterrupted.

If in doubt discuss this with a doctor or nurse. Obviously you must omit the 'dummy' inactive tablets if postponing periods while on an ED version of a phasic pill.

All in all, from body chemistry research and from the

practical point of view it is clear that phasic pills are not necessarily ideal. Yet they do form a useful addition to the available range.

Which pill should be chosen?

Even if you have been on one of the brands above half-way on one of the ladders in Figure 17 for years with no problems, I would recommend *discussing with your doctor* whether it might not now be better to try taking a pill from a lower 'rung' with a lower dose or possibly one from ladders A, B, or C using a new progestogen. Obviously many people are reluctant to 'change a winning team' but, provided you follow the instructions on page 72, you will be quite safe from pregnancy during the change-over and later. You might also even notice that some mild symptoms you have lived with on the previous pill will now improve.

The only likely problem you may run into with an ultra-low-dose pill like this is a slightly irregular bleeding pattern. This is usually only for the first two or three months while your body is getting used to it.

Can there be good reasons for not being on a below-the-lines pill in Figure 17?

Yes: not every woman is suited by one of these ultra-low-dose pills. There is that reduced 'margin for error' which means that they may not be good for those who often forget to take tablets (see page 47); nor for those who have to take interfering drugs or who may have absorption problems. Poor absorption is relatively common among women in less developed countries (page 148). And some ordinary pill-users find difficulty in obtaining a good regular bleeding pattern with the lowest-dose brands. One containing more of either hormone may then be prescribed (see below).

As all these examples have in common the fact that the blood level of the pill hormones is likely to be a little reduced, from your body's point of view it is possible (though not certain in every case) that this is almost the same thing as being on one of the ultra-low-dose pills. The situation is roughly equivalent to climbing up a moving staircase which is going down.

Tailoring the pill to you

Doctors have in the past produced elaborate schemes from which they claimed to be able to choose the right pill for each woman's hormonal make-up. Unfortunately, they never really worked, chiefly because of too little information on the effects of different formulas; and also because of the variation between women, in the way their bodies absorb and react to the pill's hormones. For example, complaints like nausea, vomiting, breast discomfort, menstrual cramps, and delay in return of periods post-pill, all tend to be commoner in underweight women. (Though weight is not otherwise a useful guide as to how strong a pill to give.)

Regardless of weight, on comparing different women at a set time after taking the same brand of tablet very different blood levels have been found. Levels of the progestogens and of the ethinyloestradiol can vary tenfold between women. Furthermore, relatively high levels of hormone (in this case the oestrogen) have been found in those pill-takers who developed high blood pressure. A likely conclusion is that many unwanted effects, both serious and 'minor', are connected with having unnecessarily high blood levels: caused either by unusually efficient absorption or inefficient elimination of the hormones. Since it is impractical to measure blood levels routinely, and low levels do have the problem of causing irregular bleeding (page 155), doctors have tended in the past to give some women more hormone than might have been necessary. In the light of the new data here and elsewhere in this new edition, I am now recommending a new policy. In general, and there are exceptions, *new prescriptions should start with a brand of pills from at or near the bottom of one of the ladders* (but not normally Loestrin 20, as its oestrogen dose is too low for acceptable control of the bleeding cycle). This policy will avoid giving any woman who tends to have high blood levels a stronger pill than the lowest available—which would be more

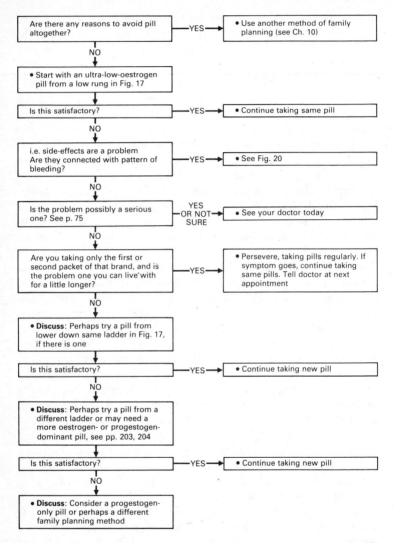

Fig. 19 Which pill?

Notes: 1. 'Discuss' means *discuss at next visit with doctor or nurse: they will not take kindly to being told by you what to do next.*

2. If moving down a ladder, start the new packet without any break.

than enough for her! Those with low levels should still receive adequate protection against pregnancy, but will be prone to problems with the bleeding pattern. These can be managed, like other side-effects, by *forewarning*, and by following the scheme of Figure 19. Note carefully the footnotes to Figure 19 and be tactful as you DISCUSS the next move with your doctor!

Which first pill?

The normal first choices in 1991 are low on one of the ladders: commonly Marvelon or Mercilon, Minulet/Femodene, Trinordiol/Logynon, Trinovum or Brevinor/Ovysmen. Smokers and others with risk factors should usually receive a pill with a lipid-friendly progestogen. But there must be flexibility (page 196). In particular, some women know themselves to be forgetful. Others will not tolerate or will become confused by *any* irregular bleeding. These may well be better off if given a slightly stronger brand from the outset.

Commonly the first choice will prove satisfactory, long term. A given brand should normally be given at least two months' trial—see Figures 19 and 20a. But if symptoms are troublesome come back as soon as necessary to discuss the next move:

If the first pill does not suit, which should be the second choice?

(a) *Problems with the bleeding cycle—bleeding on days of pill-taking*. Please look at Figure 20a and follow the questions and suggestions down the left-hand side. If you started taking the pill just after an abortion or miscarriage, the bleeding could have a special cause and you should turn at once to page 58. Otherwise one reason for this so-called 'breakthrough' bleeding is that there is too low a level of pill hormones in your blood, and therefore too little is reaching the lining of the uterus. If you do not lengthen your pill-free time (page 62) contraception should be maintained. But if you have been late in taking pills recently, or had a stomach upset, then you should follow the rules in Figures 11 and 12 (pages 61, 66–7). See also the text that goes with the figures, and pages 69–72 if there is the possibility that another drug is interfering with the pill's actions.

If you are only taking the first or second packet of pills, it is

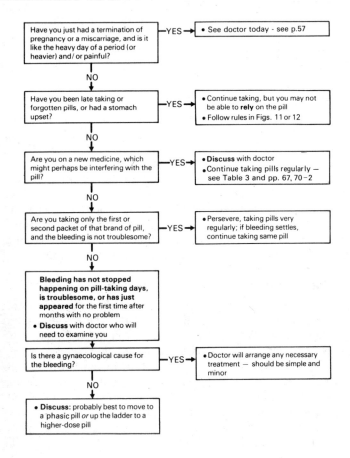

● **Bleeding on days of pill-taking**
  (i.e. 'breakthrough' bleeding)

Have you just had a termination of pregnancy or a miscarriage, and is it like the heavy day of a period (or heavier) and/or painful?	—YES→	● See doctor today - see p.57

NO ↓

Have you been late taking or forgotten pills, or had a stomach upset?	—YES→	● Continue taking, but you may not be able to **rely** on the pill ● Follow rules in Figs. 11 or 12

NO ↓

Are you on a new medicine, which might perhaps be interfering with the pill?	—YES→	● **Discuss** with doctor ● Continue taking pills regularly — see Table 3 and pp. 67, 70–2

NO ↓

Are you taking only the first or second packet of that brand of pill, and the bleeding is not troublesome?	—YES→	● Persevere, taking pills very regularly; if bleeding settles, continue taking same pill

NO ↓

Bleeding has not stopped happening on pill-taking days, is troublesome, or has just appeared for the first time after months with no problem
● **Discuss** with doctor who will need to examine you

↓

Is there a gynaecological cause for the bleeding?	—YES→	● Doctor will arrange any necessary treatment — should be simple and minor

NO ↓

● **Discuss:** probably best to move to a phasic pill *or* up the ladder to a higher-dose pill

Fig. 20a Which pill? Bleeding patterns

Note: See Figure 19 Note 1.

200   Who for the pill, and which pill?

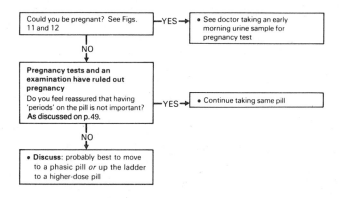

● **No bleeding at all during pill-free week** (no 'periods') – at least two missed*

Could you be pregnant? See Figs. 11 and 12	—YES→	• See doctor taking an early morning urine sample for pregnancy test

NO ↓

Pregnancy tests and an examination have ruled out pregnancy Do you feel reassured that having 'periods' on the pill is not important? **As discussed on p.49.**	—YES→	• Continue taking same pill

NO ↓

• **Discuss**: probably best to move to a phasic pill *or* up the ladder to a higher-dose pill

Fig. 20b Which pill? Bleeding patterns

* Very important: If only one 'period' missed and there is no reason to suspect failure of the pill, do not delay—start the next cycle of pills on the usual day (see page 66).

well worth persevering as improvement can be expected. Otherwise—and whenever bleeding is a persistent or unexplained problem, or occurs with love-making—you should see your doctor soon. There are some rare gynaecological causes for bleeding which he needs to eliminate by examining you. One example would be a polyp at the entrance to the uterus. Ectopy (page 119) can very occasionally cause some kind of bleeding too. Any treatment necessary should be simple and minor, often just as an out-patient.

But usually there is no gynaecological explanation. The problem can then often be solved by using a phasic pill, pages 192–5; or otherwise by moving up the ladder to another pill which contains the same hormones as the one which you are presumably finding satisfactory in other ways. For example, if you were to develop 'breakthrough' bleeding or spotting with Ovysmen or Brevinor in ladder E your doctor might suggest Norimin/Neocon. If necessary you could even go up more rungs on the same ladder to Norinyl-1 or Ortho-Novin 1/50.

(b) *Problems with the cycle—no bleeding during the pill-free week*. You should now refer to Figure 20b. Have you forgotten any pills? Or has something else happened recently which might reduce your protection against pregnancy? If there is any doubt pregnancy must be ruled out by one or perhaps a series of urine tests and probably an examination (see page 66). If you start getting symptoms such as nausea or miss two periods in a row it is vital to have a pregnancy test even if no pills were missed.

Once the explanation of pregnancy has been ruled out, then you may like to stop and think whether it really bothers you whether you get bleeding between packets of pills or not. The fact is that no pill-user ever has real *periods* anyway. The bleeding which you think of as a period is entirely artificial (page 47) and caused by you when you stop taking pills for seven days in each 28 days. If the loss of the pill hormones does not cause a bleed, it just means there was no blood to come away. So far as we know either no bleeding, or the passing of a little dark-brown discharge rather than blood, mean nothing as far as your health is concerned; nor do they indicate any risk to your future fertility (see page 127). In fact, if you were to transfer to another method, I can almost guarantee that your periods would come back with no more delay than that experienced by the average pill-user.

If this reassures you, you could, if you wish, stay on the same pill more or less indefinitely. Otherwise the situation once again, with the approval of your doctor, may be to try first a phasic pill and then perhaps the brand on the next available rung up your particular ladder. In summary, the last six pages are about

> *giving each woman the lowest dose which the woman finds acceptable, because it is just—but only just—enough to stop her womb bleeding on the 'wrong' days.*

Obviously this dose may be different for different women.

What about side-effects which are nothing to do with the bleeding pattern?

Please refer now to the bottom half of Figure 19. If you have a symptom which could perhaps be serious (see the list on page 75), or if you are not quite sure that it is *not* one of those, you should contact your doctor today and take no further pills unless the doctor says that you may. If it is a less serious side-effect such as gain in weight, unpredictable headaches which are not migraines, or breast symptoms; and if it continues beyond the two or three courses of pills which are necessary to give your body a chance to get used to any particular brand, then there are two possibilities. First, you could move further down your current ladder provided there is a pill brand available which contains even less hormone. NB *Always follow the rules on page 71 if going down a ladder.*

Secondly, if there is no room for you to go down any more rungs on a particular ladder, or it seems possible that your side-effect is due to a particular progestogen, then the other 'trial-and-error' possibility to discuss with your doctor is a 'sideways shift'. This means moving to a different ladder altogether and taking a pill which contains a different progestogen combined with the oestrogen.

More specifically, there are some guidelines which may sometimes be helpful in deciding which of the two hormones in the pill is the one whose dose should be lowered the most:

(a) *Conditions linked with relative oestrogen excess may be helped by a more* PROGESTOGEN-DOMINANT *pill*
    nausea
    dizziness
    symptoms of tension/irritability
    feelings of bloating/cyclical weight gain due to fluid retention
    vaginal discharge (no infection present)
    some cases of breast tenderness with enlargement
    growth of breast lumps (pages 132, 142)
    growth of fibroids (pages 121–2)
    endometriosis (page 122)
For any of the above problems it is often worth trying a progestogen-dominated pill—i.e. one with the lowest possible dose of oestrogen combined with *relatively* more progestogen. Lowering the oestrogen (e.g. Mercilon) is usually preferable to raising the progestogen (as in Eugynon 30/Ovran 30), for the

reasons discussed on pages 154–6, but Loestrin 30 is the acceptable first choice if that is necessary.

 (b) *Conditions linked with relative progestogen excess may be helped by a more* OESTROGEN-DOMINANT *pill.*

 some cases of sustained weight gain
 some cases of depression/tiredness
 loss of sex urge (libido)
 dryness of vagina
 acne, and greasiness of skin and head hair
 unwanted hair growth (hirsutism)

For these problems the most oestrogen-dominant pills are the first ones *above the top line* in each of the ladders D and E. Severe acne may need 50 mcg oestrogen for best results. But, on the general principle of lowering the total dose of hormone given, among the ultra-low combined pills the most oestrogen-dominant formulae are Ovysmen/Brevinor, Marvelon, and Femodene/Minulet. There is also available in some countries under the brand name Dianette or Diane 35 a pill containing a particular progestogen with strong anti-androgenic effects in the body, cyproterone acetate, combined with 35 mcg of ethinyl-oestradiol. This is recommended chiefly for the (very effective) *treatment* of severe acne and hirsutism, but it is *also* an effective contraceptive.

Fortunately, most women find the first pill they try is satisfactory.

Are all side-effects actually caused by the treatment received?

In one very interesting research study from Mexico, 147 women who had recently had a miscarriage and did not mind too much when they again became pregnant were given tablets which they thought were some kind of contraceptive. In fact, however, they were all given nothing more than *placebos* (dummy tablets of milk-sugar plus starch). These 147 women were then followed for a total of 424 woman-months. During only one-third of these months of observation were there no symptoms reported. Decreased libido was reported in 30 per cent of the months; dizziness in 11 per cent; indeed no less than 31 different effects of the 'no treatment' were reported!

Similar results were obtained in studies in which the pill was compared with dummy tablets without the women knowing which they were receiving. (They were using another method as their contraceptive.) Other studies in which placebo tablets were used in comparison with other drugs, and where the volunteers were men, have similarly shown that dummies can 'cause' numerous symptoms.

The reason for referring to this research is not to say women imagine the problems they have with the pill, which can be real enough as already described in this book. However it must be clear that the pill could sometimes be blamed for things which are not really caused by any effects of its hormones. If women are very anxious about possible health risks of taking the pill, or if their doctor or nurse is in a hurry and fails to inspire them with any confidence, it seems that they are more likely to complain of such problems as dizziness, headaches, and mild depression. On the other hand, researchers have shown that women who do not often complain of nervous symptoms, or who are prescribed the pill by somebody who answers their questions and is reassuring and checks by examining them that all is well, are much less likely to complain of symptoms from the pill, to keep changing brands, or to discontinue it altogether.

In the RCGP Study no less than 27 per cent of the pill-users stopped the method in the first year while still feeling the need for contraception. No fewer than 199 symptoms or diseases were given as the reason for giving up the pill, and in only a small fraction is there any convincing evidence of them being a true effect of the pill. A further very relevant fact is that about one in five of these women who stopped the pill while still planning to continue avoiding pregnancy in fact became pregnant within the next year. Perhaps more should have considered:

The mini-pill or progestogen-only pill

This is the place to look in detail at this completely different pill which contains no oestrogen at all. It can be a logical choice especially:

(i) if reducing the health risk of your method to the absolute minimum is particularly important to you;

(ii) if you are a woman with a relative contra-indication to the combined pill from the list on pages 177–82;

(iii) if you have a side-effect problem which has not been dealt with by following the suggestions of Figure 19.

Turn to the next chapter and the secrets of this now more popular kind of pill will be revealed.

8

....

The progestogen-only pill
(mini-pill)

What are mini-pills?

First let us be clear what they are not. They are not low-dose combined oral contraceptives or COCs for short, which have been the subject of most of this book so far. Even ultra-low-dose combined pills still contain both the hormones oestrogen and progestogen. Mini-pills represent a completely different method of contraception.

Because the word 'mini-pill' causes so much confusion, I shall just label them progestogen-only pills or POPs for short.

Unlike combined pills, POPs are taken every day while contraception is needed, including during periods. They contain no oestrogen and the progestogen itself is generally also in a lower dose than in combined pills. So it is believed that POPs are even less likely to harm your health than COCs. Note carefully that though this is a reasonable belief, it has not been *proved* true. POPs have not been used by enough women for long enough for the possible medium- to long-term unwanted effects to show up. Overall they have not yet been studied nearly as thoroughly as the combined pills. However, it is known that, like them, an overdose of POPs can cause no serious harm to an average adult or child.

How do they work?

You will find it helpful to refer to Table 11. It shows that POPs do not depend on stopping release of the egg. As a result, most periods that a woman gets on this pill, unlike those on the COC

Table 11 How progestogen-only pills prevent pregnancy
(The more +s means the greater the effect)

	'Ordinary' combined pills	Progestogen-only mini-pills
1. Reduced FSH therefore follicles stopped from ripening and egg from maturing	++++	++
2. LH surge stopped so no egg-release	++++	++
3. Cervical mucus changed into a barrier to sperm	+++	+++
4. Lining of uterus made less suitable for implantation of an embryo	+++	++(+)
5. Uterine tubes perhaps affected so that they do not transport egg so well (uncertainty about this)	+	+·
Expected pregnancy rate per 100 women using the pill method for one year (compare use of NO METHOD = 80–90)	0.2 to 1	0.3 to 5

Notes: The combined pill is *very* reliable with plenty of back-up effects—but relies chiefly on effects 1 and 2.

The progestogen-only pill is thought to rely chiefly on effect 3. Egg-release is disturbed or stopped in over half of all POP-users, increasingly with increased duration of use.

(page 47), are natural ones. They are due to the loss of the natural progesterone and oestrogen from the ovary reaching the lining of the uterus, as the corpus luteum comes to the end of its usual limited life span—about two weeks after egg-release.

So POPs operate by interfering with the passage of sperm through the mucus at the entrance to the uterus (cervix). The slippery mucus which is normally released under the influence of oestrogen is altered by the artificial progestogen and becomes a scanty and thick material which is an effective barrier to the sperm. This happens whether or not the POP prevents egg-release that month. One way of looking at this is to *consider the POP as a barrier method of family planning which is taken by mouth.*

The POP method does also interfere with egg-release, especially in long-term use and among older users. When this happens it makes the method even more effective, of course, but it also causes erratic bleeding patterns—especially complete absence of the periods (see below).

How effective are POPs?

If taken very regularly they are capable of giving protection second only to the combined pill. The failure rate is about 0.3 to 5 per 100 woman-years. See page 47 for what this means. There is a definite suggestion in some of the research that the POP like other progestogen-only methods may be less likely to fail in thin women, but do less well among the overweight. Even more important is the efficiency of the user and how fertile she is. The lowest failure rate is in older women (over 35)—indeed over 40 it really is just as safe as the combined pill.

This pill is therefore especially suitable for an older or less fertile woman who is a really good pill-taker. You should discuss the pros and cons with your doctor.

How are POPs taken?

The answer is: every single day, 365 days a year, at the same time of day, and whether or not you are having any kind of bleeding that day. In the last chapter I pointed out that the ultra-low-dose COCs of Table 9 (pages 186–7) are very effective but may have a slightly reduced margin for error. This is even more true of the progestogen-only pills. They can be at least as reliable as an IUD, and perhaps more so if taken with the regularity of clockwork at exactly the same time each day.

How should POPs be taken?

The sperm-barrier effect on the cervical mucus mentioned just now reaches its maximum about four or five hours after each pill is taken. As the commonest time for love-making is around bedtime, the very best time to take the pill can be in the early evening, say at 7 o'clock. This is not to say that if you fancy sex at breakfast-time or in the middle of the afternoon you will not be protected. Once you are fully established on the POP you should have quite adequate protection at any time in the 24 hours. It is just logical to have the best possible protection around the most common time for your own love-making. There could of course be problems if your partner is on night-duty or if you are: you just have to work things out between you!

This argument means that *for most women the very worst time to take their POP is bedtime* because they are then regularly relying on the mucus effect from the pill taken 24 hours earlier. So pill-taking at breakfast or lunch-time would be better and indeed perfectly acceptable. More important than the precise time is the regularity with which you take your pill at the same hour of each day. Yet it is not as reliable as the COC, so no one can promise you *complete* security against pregnancy even if you are obsessionally regular in your pill-taking.

How do I start taking this pill?

You take your first tablet on the first day of *your next period*, and start each subsequent packet immediately following the last tablet of the previous one. Because the full effects shown in Table 11 take some time to build up, it used to be said 'you do not rely on this pill until you have taken it for 14 days'—implying a method like the sheath during that time. This is now held to be too cautious, see Important Note, page 211. Similarly, no extra precautions are required if the POP is started on the day of a *miscarriage* or *termination of pregnancy*.

After *delivery of a baby*, this pill does not increase the risk of blood clots. So it *can* be started as early as the seventh day. However extra bleeding or spotting can be caused by an early start even in breast-feeders, so like the COC it is usually better to start in the fourth week. No extra precautions are required if you prefer to delay starting the POP until the fourth week after the birth. So long as you start no later than that, this applies even if you do not breast-feed. Another option: if periods have not yet returned, and another pregnancy has been ruled out as the cause, start the POP any time. In that case allow one week (some would say just two days) before unprotected intercourse occurs.

From and to the combined pill

1. *From the COC to the POP*. Take the first pill from the POP packet the day after the last combined pill. As there is some 'carryover' of the latter's contraceptive effects, it is then unnecessary to use another method initially as well.

2. *From the POP to the COC*, or another family planning method. It is best to have the first packet of the combined pill ready, and to transfer directly to it on the first or second day of your next definite period, perhaps before you have finished the final POP packet. This is also the best time to stop if you are transferring to a method like the sheath or the cap. The reason is that waiting to the end of your POP packet might coincide with egg-release, at the most fertile time two weeks before the next period—not a good time for changing methods.

If you do not see any periods (see below) then you could wait until the end of your current packet before taking the first COC, or starting another new method. Either way you can assume continuous protection against pregnancy.

What if I forget to take a POP?

This pill is not for the forgetful. The rules are stricter than with the COC. Please study Figure 21 carefully.

If you are more than *3 hours* late in taking the pill, then you should take the one you have missed but *use another method for two whole days (48 hours) after the pill was forgotten*. Should you have *a vomiting attack starting within 3 hours, similar loss of protection must be assumed*. See the figure for details. Diarrhoea on its own is no problem unless it is exceedingly severe (as for the COC, page 69).

Important Note: The 2-day part of the rule just given is new, and replaces the former 14-day rule for the POP. The most important contraceptive effect, on the mucus (Table 11), takes only a few hours to build up. Personally I therefore favour this 2-day rule, which is now recommended by the British FPA (since 1986).

The effectiveness of the POP can be regained quickly: but

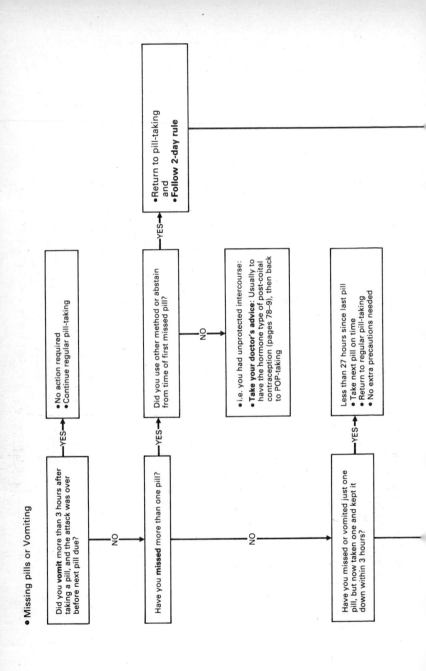

● Missing pills or Vomiting

Did you vomit more than 3 hours after taking a pill, and the attack was over before next pill due?

→ YES → ● No action required
● Continue regular pill-taking

↓ NO

Have you missed more than one pill?

→ YES → Did you use other method or abstain from time of first missed pill?

→ YES → ● Return to pill-taking and
● **Follow 2-day rule**

→ NO → ● i.e. you had unprotected intercourse:
● **Take your doctor's advice:** Usually to have the hormone type of post-coital contraception (pages 78–9), then back to POP-taking

↓ NO

Have you missed or vomited just one pill, but now taken one and kept it down within 3 hours?

→ YES → Less than 27 hours since last pill
● Take next pill on time
● Return to regular pill-taking
● No extra precautions needed

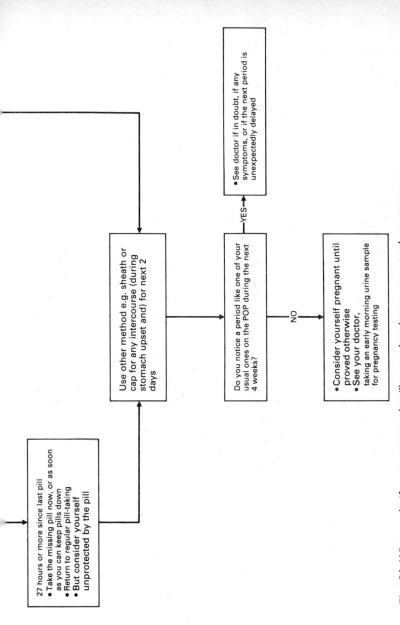

27 hours or more since last pill
- Take the missing pill now, or as soon as you can keep pills down
- Return to regular pill-taking
- But consider yourself unprotected by the pill

Use other method e.g. sheath or cap for any intercourse (during stomach upset and) for next 2 days

Do you notice a period like one of your usual ones on the POP during the next 4 weeks?

YES

- See doctor if in doubt, if any symptoms, or if the next period is unexpectedly delayed

NO

- Consider yourself pregnant until proved otherwise
- See your doctor, taking an early morning urine sample for pregnancy testing

Fig. 21 What to do if progestogen-only pills are taken late or a stomach upset occurs

Note: The 2-day rule is new. See Important Note, page 211.

The progestogen-only pill 213

there is no doubt that it is less than that of the combined pill, and it is also *losable much more rapidly—within 3 hours in fact.* No change there. In fact, post-coital contraception may be advised if you have taken a risk having missed two or more POPs—see pages 78–9.

What about interactions between the POP and other medicines?

The POP has never been widely enough used for us to be able to answer some of the questions about it—and this is one of them. We have to assume that *except for certain of the antibiotics*, those medicines that can affect the COC also reduce the effectiveness of the POP. See the discussion on pages 67–72 and Table 3. So extra precautions need to be used during short courses of treatment (and for 48 hours thereafter). The POP is not normally considered reliable enough against pregnancy when used long term, for example, by women with epilepsy who have to be on a drug from Table 3. But if nothing else suits it has been suggested that three or even four POP tablets a day might be enough to restore effectiveness. The POP probably does not interfere with the action of other medicines to any important extent.

In all these circumstances—missing pills, stomach upsets (vomiting or diarrhoea), the use of interfering drugs—your loss of protection against pregnancy is more likely and more immediate than with the combined pill. You are also more likely to get irregular bleeding which is in any case a commoner problem on the POP.

What if I am late for a period?

As a general rule on this pill, whatever your periods do, coming early or late, or not at all, do not stop taking the tablets unless advised to do so by a doctor. Irregular bleeding and no bleeding are the main side-effects. But if you go six weeks with no period, and especially if you see no bleeding during the four weeks after pills have been missed or after a stomach upset, you do need to arrange a pregnancy test on an early morning specimen of your urine, to be on the safe side. See again Figure 21. It is especially important to arrange this test and see your doctor if you get symptoms like early morning nausea. If the result is negative you should take your doctor's advice as to whether and how often it should be repeated: no need of course if you then get a period. If the test shows you are pregnant you should stop taking the pill. If pregnancy is extremely likely because you have missed more than one pill while taking no other precautions (see Figure 21), your doctor may well advise you at an earlier stage to stop the method. In fact the tiny dose of progestogen in the POP is even less likely than the ordinary pill to harm an early pregnancy (see page 130). But it is better to play safe, using another kind of contraception until you know for sure.

What if I continue with no periods and am shown not to be pregnant?

This is rather more complicated. In some women, even the small amount of hormone present in the POP can be enough to stop egg-release. This means two things: first, the base of the brain and pituitary gland are being made inactive by this low dose of a single hormone in the same way as happens in any woman who is taking any 'ordinary' combined pill. *So no egg-release means you are as protected against pregnancy as if you were on the combined pill.* But second, *on the progestogen-only pill, no egg-release means no periods.* Why not? The reason of course is that on the POP you do not (*and must not*) take the pills in a cyclical way, with the regular 7-day break in each 28 days. That is what causes the 'periods' on the ordinary pill (see pages 47–9). They are quite artificial, caused by the pill hormones acting directly on the lining of the uterus, and should really be called 'hormone withdrawal bleeds'.

If then you get no periods at all on the POP no eggs are being released: so you are actually much better protected from pregnancy than any friend of yours also using this pill who goes on seeing regular periods and is therefore being continually reassured!

Of course this is only true if you continue to be unfailingly regular in taking your pills, and even then only if tests and perhaps an examination have proved that the method has not let you down. It is a bit muddling that the same situation—i.e. absence of periods—could mean *either* that you are already pregnant *or* that you are extra safe against pregnancy! It can also be rather worrying and is one of the problems of the POP method. As usual, if in doubt, discuss the next step with your doctor.

How reversible is the POP?

As the dose of hormone is so low, the fertility of a woman after stopping this pill is believed to be the same as it would have been at her age if she had never taken it. Remember though that at least one in 10 of all couples experience delay or may need some treatment before they achieve a pregnancy.

If while taking the POP you went on seeing periods, this is almost a test of fertility as it probably means that in spite of taking the artificial hormone you were able to continue to have egg-release and natural periods.

What, however, if while taking the POP you have no periods at all? Well, all this means *if you are shown not to be pregnant* is that while on the POP your own menstrual cycle has been in the same 'resting' situation as it is in any *average* woman taking the ordinary COC. The POP has done the same temporary inactivating job on the base of your brain, pituitary gland, and ovaries as the combined pill does to everybody: no less, and *no reason* to suppose more. This pill does after all contain only a very small amount of a single hormone. So there is a very good chance that when you discontinue taking the POP your periods and fertility will be the same as they would have been at your current age had you never taken a single pill.

You could of course test the point about your periods by using a barrier method instead for two or three months, like the sheath or the cap. Some doctors would be prepared to allow you to transfer to one of the lowest-dose COCs available. This will give regular, reassuring, withdrawal bleeds. But remember these are not important—and you will now be taking a larger dose of hormones than has proved to be strictly necessary to stop egg-release in your case. So some women prefer simply to continue taking the POP, long term, despite seeing no periods.

If after stopping *either* the progestogen-only pill *or* the COC or any other method your periods do not return for six months or more, this is a different matter. The cause should be sought by appropriate examinations and tests (see page 77).

What about side-effects of the POP?

We still know far too little about these, especially any long-term effects, but what we do know is reassuring when compared with our knowledge about the combined pill.

* Research into *body chemistry*. The factors involved in blood clotting seem to be quite unaffected on the POP. They also return to normal if a woman transfers to it from the combined pill. But the Glucose Tolerance Test mentioned on page 87 is minimally changed in POP-users, and there are very slight changes in the blood levels of the hormone insulin and in blood fats (lipids). Some studies suggest that these particular tests are actually even less affected by some 'bottom-of-the-ladder' COCs in Figure 17 (pages 190–1). In other words the oestrogen in those can cancel out some of the effects of the progestogen on body chemistry, as discussed on pages 154–6. But the same oestrogen has other snags which are very well established (especially its effects on clotting factors). So the picture is confused at present. What we badly need is a *POP which uses one of the new lipid-friendly progestogens (pages 155–6)*.

Blood pressure. Overall blood pressure tends to be *much* less affected than on the combined pill. It often falls on transferring from the COC to the POP.

In general the systems of the body seem to be affected less by this pill than by even the lowest-dose COCs in Figure 17. Part of the reason may be that the woman's own ovary carries on producing at least some oestrogen, which counteracts unwanted effects of the (albeit tiny) dose of progestogen.

So the POP is an excellent pill and would be much more widely used if only it did not tend to cause an *erratic bleeding pattern*. Although the periods which happen are caused the normal way (page 207), the progestogen can, and often does, modify a POP-user's cycle, and affect the bleeding mechanisms of the lining of the uterus. So, on the one hand, as already explained, there may be complete absence of bleeding for months on end. On the other hand, periods can be more frequent; longer or shorter than before; very irregular; or relatively regular with frequent and unexpected extra bleeds from the lining of the uterus in between the periods. This is the major problem of the method. But forewarned is forearmed and many women adjust very well after a month or two to their new bleeding pattern. Other symptoms of the menstrual cycle, such as *pre-menstrual tension*, are very variable, depending on how much the cycle is altered by the POP. They are usually unchanged but in different women they can be worsened or improved! In the Oxford/FPA Study more women stopped the POP for *breast tenderness* than stopped the COC for that reason.

A much smaller proportion of women than is found on the combined pill complain of things like *weight gain*, *loss of libido*, *headaches*, and *dizziness*. As with the COC, these symptoms are usually only a problem in the first two or three months and it is worth persevering at least that long as they could well disappear. A few women also complain of pain caused by *cysts on the ovary* of the type described on page 123, though more often such cysts give no symptoms. Far from protecting against these as the COC does, the POP actually makes them more likely to be formed.

Finally, like the IUD, if a pregnancy does occur during use of the POP it seems it may be more likely to be in the wrong place: particularly in the uterine tube. This is known as an *ectopic pregnancy*. This is a rare complication, occurring in about one in 1,000 POP-users per year in a country like Britain: but it is serious as the pregnancy cannot continue normally. Eventually it may break into a blood-vessel. As this could lead to internal bleeding an emergency operation is usually essential.

The main reason for all ectopics is damage to a tube by previous infection, most commonly with chlamydia (page 25). Since on the POP (unlike the COC) egg-release can still occur, a sperm may manage to get through the barrier of altered cervical mucus; and then because of the damaged tube the fertilized egg may get held up and grow there rather than on the wall of the uterus. Whatever the explanation, in practice this means that if while on the POP you start to have an increasingly severe pain in the lower abdomen, usually on one side or the other, and not coming and going like normal menstrual cramps, then you should be seen and *examined* by a doctor. If the cause is an ectopic, the period will generally be a few days overdue, or you may have had what seemed like a prolonged and lighter-than-usual period. However, even without this, when in doubt you should see a doctor promptly. If he or she feels it possible that you have a pregnancy in the tube—it can often be very difficult to be sure—then you will be referred to the nearest hospital for further tests and possibly an operation if required.

Who should avoid the POP?

Here you will find it useful to refer to pages 171–7 to help you with the next statement: that absolute contra-indications to the COC are normally only relative contra-indications to the POP (reasons for extra discussion and supervision). Although there is no research that proves that *diseases of the circulation* occur on this pill more often than among non-users of pills, a past history of any of these is still described as a reason for not taking them. But many doctors including me strongly disagree with this policy for an oestrogen-free contraceptive and are prepared carefully to prescribe the POP for women who have such a past history, *unless they are at especially high risk.* Any *serious side-effect on the COC which was not clearly due to oestrogen* would mean also avoiding the POP in future. Undiagnosed bleeding or possible pregnancy are other exclusions, at least until they are properly diagnosed.

An extra reason for usually avoiding the POP would be any *history of an ectopic pregnancy*—see above. As that rare complication reduces fertility (and also because of the higher failure rate of POPs, page 209), younger women who want a family in due course are normally advised to take the COC as first choice over the POP. But the latter is still a good second choice.

If *cysts of ovarian follicles* (page 123) have caused pain in the past, the COC is preferable to the POP.

Since it contains no oestrogen, the POP does not have to be stopped during immobilization or before major surgery.

Which variety of POP should I choose?

The kinds available in Britain are as shown in Table 12, and also in Figure 17 in the last chapter, where they are shown as at 'ground level', because they contain so little hormone. If you live in another country, refer again to the World directory of pill names (page 301) to discover how the locally available brands of POP are related to those shown here.

Any of these pills may prove satisfactory. If you develop a problem with the cycle or any other side-effect with one POP, and still wish to use the method, then it is certainly worth switching to one of the others. At the moment this has to be done very much on a trial-and-error basis. If you persevere, the menstrual pattern normally becomes acceptable after a few months. If you get no periods at all, and this is shown not to be due to pregnancy, there is often no medical objection to your continuing the same POP.

One day we will hopefully have a POP which uses one of the now preferred 'lipid friendly' progestogens (pages 155–6).

Who might consider using the POP?

The short answer is, anyone above the age of about 25 who is considering taking a pill at all. This would be the obvious choice if maximum safety against health risk is particularly important to you. You will be losing a bit in effectiveness as compared with the combined pill: but not too much if you are good at remembering to take pills, especially if you are over 35 (page 209). A lot may depend on how well you manage to live with an unpredictable menstrual cycle.

Because of these two snags, the POP really comes into its own when there is a *relative contra-indication* to the combined pill. This means the second list on pages 177–82 of *conditions which require special supervision* if any pill is taken. (But as noted on page 214, item 12 on that list, the long-term use of

Table 12 Brands of progestogen-only pills available in Britain

Name of pill	No. in packet	Progestogen content (mcg)	Remarks
Group D		*levonorgestrel*	
Neogest	35	37.5	Plus in addition 37.5 mcg *inactive* progestogen
Microval	35 ⎫	30	⎧ No extra, inactive, hormone
Norgeston	35 ⎭		⎨ —these are therefore
			⎩ preferred to Neogest
Group E		*norethisterone*	
Micronor	28 ⎫	350	
Noriday	28 ⎭		
Group E (cont.)		*ethynodiol diacetate*	
Femulen	28	500	

Note: Groups contain the same progestogens as the groups with the same letter in Tables 9 and 10 (pages 186–7, 188) and the ladders in Figure 17 (pages 190–1).

'interfering' drugs, would usually go against the choice of a POP.)

Out of the list, I think the POP is particularly valuable for *smokers* and for *women over the age of 35* (page 179). It is excellent for *diabetics*, both because it seems to cause less health risk and because it is extra effective as they can remember to take it so regularly with their evening insulin injection. This is the best time of day (pages 209–10). It can be tried sometimes with success in those with *blood pressure problems* on the pill. Some doctors recommend the POP for women *nearing the change of life*.

If the older POP-user has no periods, it can be quite difficult to know when the menopause actually happens, though a blood test can sometimes help. High values of the hormone FSH are to be expected if the menopause has occurred. Then the POP can be stopped and another method used for one year. If there is still no period, this is the classical way to decide that it is safe to have unprotected intercourse: but the wait can be shortened considerably if after stopping the POP 'hot flushes' occur and a repeat FSH test is high, in a woman over age 45.

If irregular bleeding occurs, particularly between periods, it may be necessary to do an out-patient womb-sampling test or less often a D & C, to be sure that there is no gynaecological problem.

Incidently, so-called hormone replacement therapy, which may be prescribed for symptoms around the menopause, should not be relied on as a contraceptive. The dose system is different from that used in any kind of contraceptive pill, and pregnancy is possible—unless of course you had definitely reached the menopause first, before the treatment started. If you need this kind of treatment before the menopause careful use of the 20 mcg oestrogen-containing pill Mercilon may be best (pages 189, 258).

If any of this applies to you and you have any queries, discuss the whole matter with your doctor or the clinic.

The commonest reason why many women choose to transfer to the POP is *because of side-effects* on the COC. Weight gain, nausea, depression, and headaches all seem to be helped by this move. Blood pressure has already been mentioned. If a combined pill-user develops chloasma, the skin pigmentation problem described on page 134, it often improves if she transfers to the POP.

Breast-feeding: the main use of the POP worldwide

This pill does not interfere at all with the quantity or significantly with the quality of breast milk. (The COC, however, sometimes does, and most doctors now feel that it is illogical to use it during breast-feeding.) A very tiny amount of the hormone in all POPs has been shown to get into the milk, the least being found in milk from women who use pills containing only levonorgestrel—i.e. Norgeston and Microval. This causes concern to some mothers. It is true that we really have no adequate knowledge of what effects the POP content of a mother's milk might have on the newborn baby. And yet, putting it the other way, there is absolutely no evidence that this amount of hormone has ever caused a baby any harm. After more than two years of full breast-feeding the infant of a mother using these POPs will have taken the equivalent of just one tablet!

To put this in perspective, if a breast-feeding woman smokes cigarettes, a far greater number of potentially dangerous chemicals are swallowed by the baby (see pages 50–1).

If you plan to feed your baby yourself—and there is abundant scientific evidence that human breast milk is better for human babies than any kind of modified cow's milk—you might discuss the use of this type of pill during the months that you are breast-feeding. Your protection against pregnancy is probably as good as that of any woman on the COC, as *full* breast-feeding supplements the contraceptive action of the POP. When you or your baby decide to cut down on the breast-feeding, and especially when your periods return, you may well prefer to change back to an ultra-low-dose combined pill from Table 9, pages 186–7. This will give extra reliability and a regular monthly 'period'. On the other hand, you may find that the POP is so satisfactory that you prefer to continue using it.

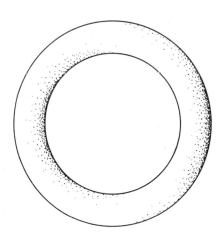

Fig. 22 The progestogen-only contraceptive vaginal ring

The progestogen-only contraceptive vaginal ring ('Femring')

This is made of a special plastic known as Silastic, see Figure 22 which shows it actual size. A steady amount of the progestogen levonorgestrel gets through the skin of the vagina directly into the bloodstream (therefore not having to go through the liver, which is an advantage, page 116). The dose is about 20 mcg a day, about the same as finally reaches the blood after a tablet of Microval or Norgeston (see Table 12) has passed through the stomach and liver.

So *in most ways this vaginal ring is like the POP*, except for where it goes—and not having to remember to take tablets every day. Practically everything earlier in this chapter about the POP is true of Femring, including the way it works to stop pregnancy, its similar effectiveness, its minimal effects on body chemistry, its advantages, and its side-effects.

If you are given Femring to try, you simply squeeze it and push it high into the vagina on the first day of your period. It slips in easier than you might expect and finds its own place (unlike the diaphragm it does not need to be in a special position related to the cervix). It can then be left for 90 days in a row, after which a new one is required to keep the hormone levels up. If preferred by either you or your partner it is good to know that you may take it out for love-making, but preferably for no more than about one hour at a time. Indeed, if you forget to put it back until three hours or more have gone by, as with the POP extra precautions are necessary for the next 48 hours: just follow the instructions in Figure 21 and on page 211. But of course there is no problem with the ring's effectiveness if you have a stomach upset—one advantage!

If it slips out in the toilet as sometimes happens, just retrieve the ring and wash it in clean water. You can then put it back for yourself. If this keeps happening you will need to discuss the situation with your doctor.

If you are overweight, meaning more than about 70 kg (11 stone) there is a strong suspicion that Femring will be less effective. So another method may be preferable: unless you have reduced fertility already (because of being above age 40 for example) or can manage to lose the excess weight . . .

The ring can sometimes cause a problem of its own: vaginal irritation or discharge. But as with the POP the commonest side effect is irregular bleeding, including seeing no periods at all. As usual, once discussed with the doctor or nurse, if the inconvenience can be lived with it does not mean any kind of health risk.

Like the POP again, the ring is not quite as effective as the combined pill for young and highly fertile women. Nor does it protect against AIDS. But all in all this is a most welcome new choice in contraception.

9

....

The future of family planning: and what became of the male pill?

It should by now be very clear that both types of pill discussed in this book leave a lot of room for improvement. What should we look for in an IDEAL future method of birth control?

Perhaps the last item in Table 13 which lists the features of the ideal contraceptive is asking for too much, but we *are* talking about the ideal! For all its faults, the pill does help women who suffer discomfort or misery from their so-called 'normal' menstrual cycles. A method which was ideal in all the main ten ways listed in the Table, such as a simple, painless, totally reversible method of female sterilization, might still leave some women less well off than on the pill, if they continued to have heavy, painful periods, pre-menstrual tension, and the like.

Table 13 Features of the ideal contraceptive

---
1. 100 per cent effective
2. 100 per cent safe, with no unwanted effects ⎰ no danger
3. 100 per cent reversible ⎱ no nuisance
4. Independent of intercourse
5. Effective after acceptable, simple, painless procedure(s), not relying on the user's memory—so the 'default state' is one of contraception
6. Reversed by a simple, painless process
7. Cheap, based on simple technology, easy to distribute
8. Independent of the medical profession
9. Acceptable to every culture, religion, and political view
10. Used by, *or* obviously visible to, the woman . . . plus, as an *optional* extra—
    • Giving the user a genuine 'bonus'—one or more *good* side-effects!

I wish it were not necessary to add number 10 to the list, but I think the point should be made. It is a sad comment on the relationship of many couples that they can share each other's bodies and yet be unable to share decisions about something so relevant as contraception . . . More specifically, some men are not trustworthy about contraception. Others are just forgetful or careless. An advantage of the sheath is that it gives visual proof that it has in fact been effectively used. If a male pill were ever available, it is not difficult to believe there might be some men who would claim to be taking it when they were not. See also pages 243–8.

A final and very important point to notice about the list is that if a future method could be devised which had all these features, it would make contraception just like conception: something entirely under the control of the couple concerned, which 'comes naturally', with no need to involve doctors or hopefully anyone else.

Why have we not yet got better methods of family planning?

This is a good question: part of the answer is that too little money and scientific effort have been put into this kind of work. Looking back it seems incredible, but family planning research did not rate at all highly; maybe this was due to hang-ups persisting from an earlier time when many people thought it was analogous to devising better methods of house-breaking, so sinful did they perceive birth control to be! See page 9. We may have come a long way since then, in our attitudes to sex and the role of women, but not far enough.

There are other reasons too why we still do not have ideal methods. Generally, in medicine, one is treating an abnormal body process, caused by disease. In trying to find a method of birth control the main action is to interfere with a *normal* body process and this means taking extra-special care. The method will be used by initially healthy women or men and should not make them unhealthy; on the other hand, it could be used by people who are already unhealthy and must not do them additional harm. It will be used in both developing and 'over-developed' countries, and may pose special and different hazards in each situation. Reproduction is a very intricate mechanism, and unwanted effects have to be looked for in the offspring as well as in the user of the method. Finally, much important research cannot be done in humans for ethical reasons, yet the animals used for testing may differ in marked and sometimes misleading ways from humans.

One hopeful line of research therefore being followed is to study men and women who are otherwise healthy but known to be infertile. If their problem could be imitated in a reversible way this could provide some useful new methods. See also pages 239–40.

This has been a difficult chapter to write. Sudden scientific breakthroughs could at any time render any list of future methods either obsolete or incomplete. What seems at the time of writing to be a promising lead, may prove in due course to be a blind alley: either because of unacceptable side-effects, or because of ineffectiveness when actually tested in human beings. So I would suggest you take more notice of general principles than of the few detailed examples there has been room to quote.

You will need to keep referring to Figure 23 which illustrates the various stages or events in reproduction at which birth control methods either now do, or one day could, operate. You will see that the various stages are numbered in the flow chart. The same numbers, within the symbols for maleness and femaleness, show where each particular process takes place on the two diagrams which illustrate male and female anatomy. The manufacture of sperm is followed by their maturing, in a very long coiled tube right beside the *testicle* known as the *epididymis*. It is only after going through this tube that the sperm are mature and able to swim vigorously to their goal. At ejaculation, the climax of intercourse, the sperm are conveyed along the *vas deferens* (vas). This process takes sperm to the base of the penis and then down the *urethra* which is the tube in the middle of the penis. From then on everything happens inside the body of the woman. The sperm have to travel from the top of the *vagina*, through the *cervix*, up through the cavity of the *uterus*, and into the *uterine tube*. Even though they matured in the epididymis, they still have not reached their full capacity for fertilizing an egg. The process called *capacitation* which finally prepares them for this occurs after the sperm get into the uterus. One only of these fully capacitated sperm enters and fertilizes the egg when they meet, usually about half-way along the tube.

You should find the rest of Figure 23 easy to follow as its stages were described in Chapter 2, but if anything is not clear, you may like to refer back to pages 39–42.

The methods—in women

As I described earlier, combined pills work chiefly at stages ♀2a and ♀2b but also at stage ♂3d (by altering the cervical mucus to block the sperm), and also at stage 7 and possibly to a minor degree at stage 5. The progestogen-only pill has effects at the same stages, but relies chiefly on ♂3d. Much research is going on to give better delivery of the hormones to the body, with two main aims: first, to reduce and make more steady the blood levels given to the whole system and their impact on the liver (which receives, all at once, a big amount of any oral dose) and second, to make the methods easier for users (e.g. so they no longer have to remember to take tablets). In fact one could say that the future of the pill is not to be a pill at all!

Injectables

Injectables are one obvious development. Already in the UK and nearly 100 other countries a progestogenic drug called Depo-Provera is widely used for contraception by injection. See page 256 for more about this useful option, and Noristerat which is similar. These bypass the liver, which is good, but the blood levels vary very much over the 12 weeks between injections. Many other compounds are now being tested, to be given by the injection route. They are mostly *progestogens*. There are monthly versions being tested by WHO which also contain an oestrogen. This helps to overcome the very irregular menstrual bleeding problem of most injectables. Tiny little polymer *micro-capsules* are used, which can be injected under the skin through an ordinary needle. It is hoped that they will give a more

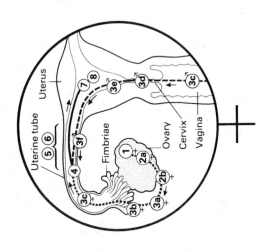

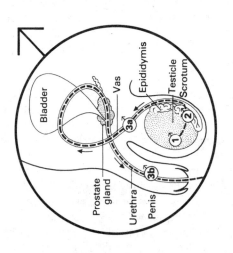

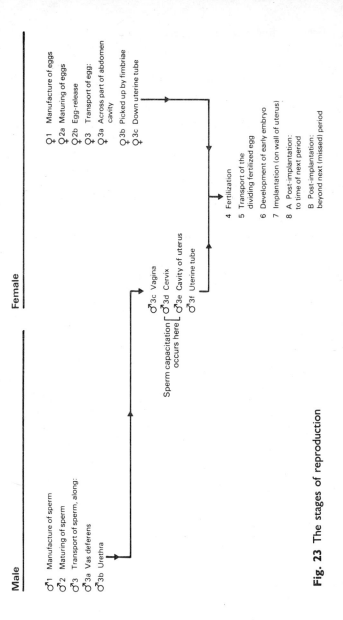

Fig. 23 The stages of reproduction

Male

♂1 Manufacture of sperm
♂2 Maturing of sperm
♂3 Transport of sperm, along:
♂3a Vas deferens
♂3b Urethra

Sperm capacitation occurs here
♂3c Vagina
♂3d Cervix
♂3e Cavity of uterus
♂3f Uterine tube

Female

♀1 Manufacture of eggs
♀2a Maturing of eggs
♀2b Egg-release
♀3 Transport of egg:
♀3a Across part of abdomen cavity
♀3b Picked up by fimbriae
♀3c Down uterine tube

4 Fertilization
5 Transport of the dividing fertilized egg
6 Development of early embryo
7 Implantation (on wall of uterus)
8 A Post-implantation: to time of next period
   B Post-implantation: beyond next (missed) period

predictable slow release of the hormones.

The major problem of all injections is that they cannot be taken out once given, if side-effects occur. So experiments are being done with removable and re-loadable *implants*. One removable type is called Norplant. These implants are inserted through small cuts in the skin under local anaesthesia and can be removed similarly, later, at the woman's request so she can conceive a baby or if there are side-effects. Norplant is nearly 100 per cent effective except in obese women for five years and fully reversible. Already available in Scandinavia it is expected on the market soon both in the USA and the UK—watch this space!

Other contraceptive delivery systems

A variety of new ways to administer contraceptive substances to the body are being tried. *Pessaries* and *sponges* to be inserted into the vagina; *rings* around the cervix within the vagina; *skin patches* and even *contraceptive bracelets* tightly applied to the skin and *nasal sprays* are some of the ideas being studied.

The vaginal rings release a progestogen, either alone or in other versions in combination with oestrogen, for absorption from the vagina. Contraception is achieved by some combination of the changes shown in Table 11, page 208, but with lower doses each day than in oral pills. All the woman has to do is to insert and remove her ring once a month or once every three months. A strong 'plus' point is that she is in complete control and can stop the method without having to see a doctor. Erratic bleeding is so far the main snag with the progestogen-only version due to come on the UK market as Femring in 1990–1. It uses levonorgestrel and has about the same effectiveness as the POP. The combined version can be thought of as 'Marvelon taken by the vagina', has been enormously popular in trials at the Margaret Pyke Centre, but will sadly not be marketed for some years.

Contraception through the nose is not such a fanciful idea as it may sound at first: the chemists have been at work on the releasing hormone (RH) which conveys the message from the base of the brain to the pituitary to cause it to release FSH and

LH (page 39). Various 'chemical cousins' (known as *analogues and antagonists*) have been produced which when sprayed into the back of the nose do seem to be able to stop the action of the normal releasing hormone on the pituitary gland, and so prevent the stages ♀2a and ♀2b of Figure 23—i.e. maturation and release of the egg. They can also be given by injection. So far they are only appropriate for use as gynaecological treatments, but that may change in time.

A lot of research is also being devoted to using *intra-uterine devices* (IUDs) to convey certain drugs. So far these have chiefly been used in an attempt to reduce the side-effects of that method, particularly pain and increased bleeding. A promising version, which should soon be marketed, is the levonorgestrel-releasing IUD. This actually *reduces* menstrual bleeding, and differs from present IUDs in another way too: evidence suggests it *protects* against pelvic infection (compare page 252). The mechanism is probably similar to that described for progestogen-containing pills (the mucus effect, page 120). Another approach to avoiding those problems is to use *intra-cervical devices* (ICDs). These are highly experimental gadgets which fit inside the passageway of the cervix. They are designed to release either a progestogen or a spermicidal substance in a slow and steady way into the passage in order to prevent sperm going any further.

IUDs work mainly at stages 4 and 7 in Figure 23. They are able to alter the interior of the uterus in such a way as to prevent the embryo from implanting. This was suspected for many years, but has been confirmed by doctors who have inserted IUDs up to five days after egg-release and found that even if the woman has had unprotected intercourse, she almost never becomes pregnant. This is therefore often used now as a 'post-coital' or emergency method (page 78).

New barrier methods

There is much interest again in these so-called 'old-fashioned' methods. This is because they are medically so safe but also because they have the potential to protect against sexually transmitted diseases including, in the case of various new designs of both *male and female condoms*, the viruses, especially HIV (see page 26). A number of types of *sponges* are being tested made of synthetic polymers, some with and some without impregnation with standard or innovative spermicides and virus-killing chemicals. So far the search for a new *cervical cap* capable of being effective when left in position long term has not been successful. One version ('Contracap') made-to-measure using the techniques dentists use and provided with a one-way valve to allow the exit of cervical mucus and menstrual blood was a heroic failure in our trials at the Margaret Pyke. Its failure rate was so high we wondered about using it in our Fertility Clinic! Win some, lose some . . . The idea is not quite dead though. Dr Kaali in New York is working on a special battery which he claims 'electrocutes' the sperm, and if (always a big if) this were found to be safe, it could be fitted in a cervical cap or other vaginal barrier.

Post-coital contraception

This term can be used for any method which is first used after intercourse, and could act from stage ♀2b (if intercourse were known to have been prior to egg-release) right through to stage 8. Existing methods include *insertion of an IUD* as just described, or the use of high doses of *oestrogen* or a combination of *oestrogen and progestogen* (page 78). As they are used no more than five days (72 hours for the hormonal methods) after intercourse, they must often work at stage 7, implantation. Current methods are not recommended on a *regular* basis: however, other substances are now being examined which may prove effective and safe enough for regular use. One is RU 486, a highly controversial anti-progestogen compound which so far is only used routinely (in France where it was discovered) for legal termination of pregnancy (stage 8B). Provided it remains under full legal and medical supervision its use in well-counselled cases at other stages in Figure 23 is in my view to be welcomed.

'Once-a-month' methods

The search is on for a method which causes the period to come on whether or not fertilization took place. Such *'once-a-month'* pills would be taken (again, there must be good legal and medical safeguards) at the expected time of the period, which is stage 8A in the Figure. Trials are in progress of RU 486 and its chemical cousins, attempting in one way or another to stop the action of progesterone from the corpus luteum. This you remember has that essential job of making sure the next period does not wash an early pregnancy away (page 37). The same result could be obtained by interfering with the ability of the early pregnancy to maintain the corpus luteum by its hormone, hCG (pages 37, 41). This looks possible by both a drug method and an immune method described below.

These and other once-a-month approaches are being researched by WHO.

Methods working at or beyond the time of the first missed period (stage 8B)

If the IUD works partly by stopping implantation (stage 7) of an already fertilized egg, and if satisfactory once-a-month methods to work at stage 8A are devised, then obviously the dividing line between contraception and abortion is becoming increasingly blurred. However, stage 8B is clearly one of early abortion, and here the *prostaglandins with or without RU 486* are already being used with some success: though there are side-effects in some cases (excessive bleeding or pain, vomiting and diarrhoea, and sometimes the need to do a D & C). There is no way that this could be recommended medically as a regular 'home' method of birth control, irrespective of the ethical aspects everyone must consider.

Ethical and moral aspects of methods operating after fertilization

Just as the definition of death has had to be altered—it is no longer cessation of the heartbeat, but death of the brain—so I think it is perhaps now out of date to say that methods which work after stage 4 (fertilization) are causing abortions. This is a very controversial area, but it seems to me that a lot of the arguments are just about definitions. I shall have to leave it to you to decide whether you do draw the line at stage 4; or else at the time of implantation (stage 7/8A). The latter will allow you to consider as contraceptives the IUD and the POP (which might occasionally, though not during breast-feeding, work by number 4 in Table 11 on page 208), as well as current post-coital pills. Points in favour of this view are: first, the *status* of the dividing fertilized egg. That is, crudely, *100 per cent certainty of non-existence* unless it can stop the next menstrual flow by getting enough hCG to the ovary—and that requires implantation (page 37). Without 'carriage', can one be 'procuring a miscarriage'? Secondly, is there logic in putting a high value on something with which nature itself is so prodigal (page 37)?

If doctors and patients are rather muddled on the subject, it is not surprising that the law in many countries is illogical and confused and the arguments often generate more heat than light! Perhaps the most important conclusion is that respect for life and a proper sense of awe about the whole process of reproduction are more important than rigid definitions.

Sterilization (stage ♂3f plus ♀3c)

If you refer to Table 13 (page 226) you will see that *female sterilization*, which prevents the sperm meeting the egg in the uterus tubes, could be ideal: if only it were even more simple and safe to perform, and if it were reversible. The latest methods of sterilization by applying clips or rings to block the tubes, often using a special telescope called the laparoscope, are already pretty good and can be done in out-patients under local anaesthetic on a walk-home basis. Some surgeons have now become so skilled in microsurgery that they can join up the ends of the tube, after cutting away the short section damaged by a clip, and claim that over 80 per cent of those re-operated on can have a baby. But this is not yet good enough: it is 'high technology' requiring much skill, and will be no help to poor people anywhere in the world.

The future may lie in some form of what is called *trans-cervical sterilization*. This means using the passageway that nature provided, through the canal of the cervix and the cavity of the uterus itself, in order to block the inner ends of the uterine tubes from within. Experiments have been carried out for some time now, with the aim of producing a cork or plug to be applied, and perhaps later removed, using another telescope instrument, the hysteroscope. Others are testing methods for applying special glues (which can stick tissues together) via the inner ends of the tubes, without using any special telescope. Even if not reversible, the prospect of doing such procedures in an out-patient clinic, with no more discomfort than the insertion of an IUD, is a welcome one—particularly for less developed countries. At the time of writing, however, there are still many technical problems.

*Immune methods

If a child is immunized against measles, an injection of a specially developed and less dangerous laboratory version of the virus causing measles is given. The child's body then produces *antibodies* which are actually special substances called immuno-globulins conveyed in the blood. The important point is that these are effective against *both* the laboratory virus *and* the natural one in the community which causes the disease. If that child is now exposed at school or anywhere to measles, the antibodies will destroy the virus. But the child can still get German measles or chicken pox, as the antibodies are, as it is called, *specific* against the one type of virus.

Now antibodies can be caused to appear not only against diseases, but also against any substances which are foreign to the body, *or* which can be altered in some subtle way so that the body treats them as though they were foreign. This can happen in an unwanted way to cause the so-called auto-immune diseases (page 137). But it also explains why it is theoretically possible to invent an immune method to work at many of the stages in Figure 23. Just one example: women could be made *immune to their husband's sperm*, and indeed this sometimes happens without being planned and causes one form of infertility. Some men develop *antibodies against their own*

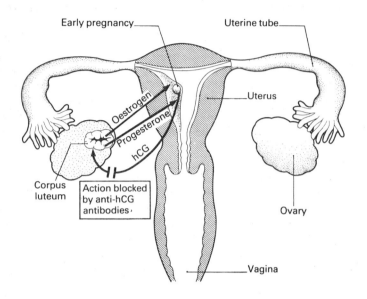

Fig. 24 An immune method: anti-hCG antibodies stop early pregnancy from maintaining corpus luteum

sperm, and although this does not always lead to them being infertile, it sometimes can do so. Again, this could lead to a male method.

There are many question marks about these methods, chiefly connected with the risk of complex antibodies being formed which might interfere with or injure other hormones, body chemicals, or tissues than those intended. However, one method, after an enormous amount of research, still appears quite promising, and is illustrated in Figure 24. The idea is to produce *a vaccine* which causes antibodies *against the hormone hCG* which was explained on pages 37, 41. This would stop the embryo 'rescuing' the corpus luteum, which it has to do if the next period is to be prevented. If this worked, the method would lead to regular periods whether or not fertilization took place. The method might even be reversible, if the job of the corpus luteum of early pregnancy could be taken over by simply giving the woman the right dose of natural oestrogen and progesterone.

Depending on their definition of an abortion, some people would have genuine misgivings about the ethics of this. There has also been a serious technical problem in that as the antibody levels fall, female animals have tended to have later abortions rather than regular bleeds seemingly like normal periods. Abortions are bad news, not only ethically and psychologically, but also because of the risk of retained products, bleeding, and infection. But the research continues.

*Blocking fertilization (stage 4)

To try to side-step these problems, researchers are now producing a vaccine whose target is the special covering of the egg known as the *zona pellucida*. This normally binds the sperm and allows just one in to fertilize the egg. Already laboratory animals have been successfully immunized, and the antibodies produced stop the sperm sticking to the zona, which therefore stops fertilization.

Whether research into these two methods, and others, will eventually lead to young women lining up for vaccination against pregnancy, in the same way as they do against measles, and whether the methods will be truly reversible, still of course remains to be seen.

Using antibodies to carry drugs to 'particular' targets in the body: so-called monoclonal antibodies can be very specific in recognizing a particular target group of cells and locating there. If the antibody could be coupled to a contraceptive drug, say, it might one day in the future be possible to ensure action only on the ovary, for example. This should virtually eliminate side-effects elsewhere.

Natural states of infertility

All women are unable to get pregnant at three main times in their lives: prior to puberty; in the earliest weeks of full breast-feeding, provided there is a very high frequency of suckling; and after the menopause. Forgetting the third state, for obvious reasons, the first two are being studied by scientists who hope to find out precisely what causes the lack of regular egg-release which prevents pregnancy at these times. A simple method of *making breast-feeding 100 per cent effective as a contraceptive* for family spacing, which it is not for most individuals in a fully predictable way, would be most valuable. Although the progestogen-only pill and the injectable Depo-Provera can be used even now, they are open to the definite objection that some of the hormone (very much more in the case of Depo-Provera than the POP) gets into the breast milk, and could harm the baby in some as yet unknown way. A method which avoids this is obviously preferable.

Natural family planning (NFP)

It would be a major advance if a method could be devised which simply and accurately predicted beforehand, and detected just afterwards, the release of the egg each month. This approach is acceptable to the Roman Catholic Church and certain other religious groups who do not accept methods which are 'artificial'. But in addition I think many other women and their partners would appreciate being able to use a simple method like the sheath or the cap just for the time when they knew, because of some simple, accurate test, that there was a chance of pregnancy. Present methods depend on calculations according to the length of previous menstrual cycles; on taking and charting the early morning temperature; and on learning to recognize certain changes in the cervical mucus which usually occur before, during, and after the fertile time. If the woman observes both mucus and temperature changes (the 'sympto-thermal' method), well-motivated couples can control their fertility well. But sooner or later many fertile long-term users even of the best existing natural family planning methods tend to be let down.

There are really two categories of NFP method. One detects egg-release, and can be quite effective (because the egg dies quickly). The other tries to predict egg-release. This is obviously more difficult, but will *always be less safe* too: because of the *remarkably good and unpredictable survival of sperm* inside the uterus (see page 8).

Ultrasound scanning—the same method that is used for checking the well-being of a baby as it grows in the uterus—can be used to watch the growth of the follicle on the active ovary, and to see the exact time of its rupture to release the egg. A really futuristic—and at present far too expensive—application of this method would be to issue women with mini-ultrasound-scan machines to be plugged into their home TVs so they could observe their own egg-release!

More practical would be a simple test of the *saliva* or *urine*. The natural LH, FSH, oestrogen, and progesterone of the menstrual cycle are excreted in the urine in a modified form, and the changing levels of these excretory products can be measured. The end-result of this research should be that a woman could test her urine every day and, according to some easily interpreted colour change, she would know exactly when her unsafe period was. For instance, she could have intercourse from the first day of her cycle just as long as the test showed 'green'. As soon as it changed to 'red', she would have to abstain or use another method. Whenever the test showed 'green' again, she could safely make love without any further precautions.

This research, which includes similar studies of saliva and of mucus, seems promising. It has the great advantage that the methods could be introduced without expensive and very time-consuming delays for safety testing which would be required for any new drug. But all these approaches are going to pose the problem that if they predict far enough ahead to allow for the most persistent surviving sperm, they may require an unpopular amount of abstinence by the couple. And like so many of the more scientifically interesting approaches in this chapter they will not protect against the virus which causes AIDS.

New methods for men

The latest development in male contraception was unveiled recently. Dr Sophie Merkin announced the preliminary findings of a study conducted on 763 male undergraduate students at a mid-West university.

The IPD (intra-penile device) resembles a tiny folded umbrella which is inserted through the head of the penis and pushed into the scrotum with a plunger-like instrument. Occasionally there is perforation of the scrotum, but this is considered insignificant since it is known that the male has few nerve endings in this area of his body. Dr Merkin declared the IPD to be statistically safe for the human male. She reported that of the 763 students tested with the device, only two died of scrotal infection, only 20 experienced swelling of the tissues, three developed cancer of the testicles, and 13 were too depressed to have an erection. She stated that common complaints ranged from cramping and bleeding to acute abdominal pains. She emphasized that these symptoms were merely indications that the man's body had not yet adjusted to the device. Hopefully the symptoms would disappear within a year.

One complication caused by the IPD and briefly mentioned by Dr Merkin was the incidence of massive scrotal infection necessitating the surgical removal of the testicles. 'But this is a rare case,' said Merkin, 'too rare to be statistically significant.' She and other distinguished members of the Women's College of Surgeons agreed that the benefits far outweighed the risks to any man.

True, this IPD is a hoax. But there is nothing like a bit of role-reversal to throw new light on old arguments. In fact, of course, the pill and other methods of family planning for women are nowhere near as dangerous and frightening as this imaginary intra-penile device. Yet some overly enthusiastic family planners in the past have sometimes talked in the same *kind* of way about the pill for women. Hence the backlash: back in the early 1960s was the pill a confidence trick by male chauvinist scientists? Was there a conspiracy, with pharmaceutical companies keen to make money, to unleash an untried chemical on the unsuspecting, docile, and passive female population?

The main point is that 'what is sauce for the goose is sauce for the gander'. In other words, if we have a pill for the goose, we surely need a pill for the gander!

Do we need a male pill?

Some women doubt whether, if a safe and effective male pill were devised, men could be trusted to take it regularly. After all, they don't 'carry the baby'. There is a powerful concept in some parts of the world, known in Latin America as 'machismo', that—quite illogically in fact—equates fertility with virility and potency. These notions seem to have influenced researchers, who have wondered whether there would be a demand for a male pill even if it were invented.

Yet the assumption that men wash their hands of birth control matters is not in fact true. It takes all types to make a world and a great many men, especially in marriage or steady relationships, show a lot more responsibility than might perhaps be expected. The best example of this is the remarkable increase in the number of vasectomy operations performed in so many countries, both developing and developed, in recent years. Men, like women, now frequently prefer their families to be small. In one survey in the US 65 per cent of the men stated that they would use a male pill or injection if it were available and not too expensive.

Research into male methods

Male contraception is biologically more difficult to achieve than female contraception. The main reason is that there is no single regular event like egg-release which can be stopped. See Figure 23. Stages ♂1 and ♂2 are continuous processes throughout a man's life from puberty to death. So instead of just stopping one egg being released about 13 times a year, we have to interfere with a process producing hundreds of millions of sperm every time a man ejaculates. Just as in the woman, any pill must not affect libido, must give extremely good protection against pregnancy, and be as free as possible from side-effects. There is a special risk here too that interference with the production of the sperm might be incomplete. So one sperm might be damaged by whatever the treatment might be, and yet manage to fertilize an egg, leading perhaps to the birth of an abnormal baby.

Yet another problem is that the manufacturing process takes a long time, about 70 days in the human male. Thus any male pill working on the manufacturing process will take at least two months to become effective. It also means that there must be a long recovery period after stopping the method. After some of the experimental methods have been stopped, some men have never got back their normal sperm counts suggesting a risk of sterility, and in others more than the usual number of abnormal sperm have been seen. So if in the recovery period another method of family planning were inadequately used, again there might be an increased risk of an abnormal baby.

Interference with the manufacturing of sperm (stage ♂1)

This can be done in two main ways, indirectly by blocking the action of the hormones from the pituitary gland which normally stimulate the process, and directly by a drug acting on the testicles.

1. *Indirect methods*. These are similar in principle to the female pill. The pituitary gland of a man produces the very same two hormones that are so important in the menstrual cycle, namely FSH and LH. However, they are not produced in a cyclical way. In a man, FSH is the hormone which is directly involved to promote sperm manufacture. LH, on the other hand, stimulates special cells, also in the testicle, which produce the male hormone, testosterone. This hormone, as well as producing the special sexual characteristics of a man such as the deepening of his voice, the hairiness of his chin, and his sex drive, joins with FSH in the business of manufacturing normal fertile sperm.

So if the levels of FSH and LH reaching the testicles can be made to drop, the process of sperm manufacture will cease. This can be done by 'negative feedback' which was explained on pages 39–40. An obvious way of doing this is to feed the man with his wife's pill! This certainly cuts down the production of FSH and LH from the pituitary and hence interferes with manufacture of sperm. Obviously, however, it is liable to interfere also with the man's masculinity. One way out of that difficulty was to use an injection which is a combination of a *progestogen with an artificial equivalent of testosterone*. This has been promising but the doses required are relatively higher than in women and there are fears about serious unwanted effects, especially on the liver.

Other indirect methods are being tried, including the use of *testosterone injections* alone; or a complex natural substance called *inhibin*. There is also the possibility of blocking the action of the releasing hormone (RH) which, as in a woman, comes down from the base of the brain to the pituitary gland and causes release of both FSH and LH. The same analogues of RH mentioned on page 233 are showing some promise, used in the male.

2. *Direct methods*. A bizarre approach has actually been tried, and that was to wrap the testicles up in warm, *woolly mufflers* made of sheepskin. This did lead to a drop in the sperm count because the sperm manufacturing process requires the testicles to be at a lower temperature than the 37°C of the rest of the body. However, this method has not been found to reduce the count predictably enough to guarantee no pregnancies. There were also some complaints that it was uncomfortable . . .

Various drugs which directly damage the manufacturing process have been tried in male animals. The experiments have had to be abandoned in most cases because they were found to be too toxic.

Sulphasalazine is a drug which has been used for years in the treatment of the disease ulcerative colitis, but was only recently found to depress sperm counts enough to be considered for testing as a male pill. Another possibility is *gossypol*. A report on the use of this substance appeared in the *Chinese Medical Journal* in November 1978. Scientific workers in Mainland China apparently discovered during the 1950s that cooking with crude cottonseed oil could lead to infertility, and it was the men that seemed to be affected. The active ingredient was tried first in a number of different experimental animals. Then 4,000 healthy men were put on regular gossypol treatment for up to four years. Close on 100 per cent of them became infertile as judged by sperm counts of zero or well below the usually accepted levels for fertility. Side-effects were said to be mild and uncommon.

So far, so good. This 'Chinese sperm take-away', as it has been called, certainly seems a promising male contraceptive. However, there have been so many disappointments in this field of research into new methods for men, that we cannot be optimistic before far more exhaustive safety checks which are being done through the World Health Orginization have been completed. Side-effects are proving more of a problem than was first suggested by the Chinese scientists. The chief one is a feeling of weakness, probably connected with a lowering of potassium in the body. Digestive disturbances and loss of sex drive are reported. And often there is such an extremely long recovery time necessary before the number and appearance of the sperm returns to normal, that doubts have been expressed about gossypol's reversibility at all in some men.

Animal research shows no effects on the hormones FSH and LH, which is good, but hamsters fail to put on weight normally when given gossypol. In summary it looks unlikely that gossypol itself will prove to be that elusive safe reversible male contraceptive. But the initial lead has been helpful, and there is hope that variants produced by the chemists may result in a product suitable for use by ordinary couples.

Maturing of the sperm in the epididymis (stage ♂2)

The epididymis is a very long (7 m), fine, coiled-up tube, which forms into something about the size of a baby's little finger closely applied to the testicle. It receives the sperm leaving the production line in the testicle and its main job is to deliver at the other end, at the start of the vas, sperm which are now mature and able to swim. Several drugs have been found to interfere with this maturing process. The great advantage of acting at this stage, if only a safe drug could be discovered, is that there would be a far more rapid loss and return of fertility than by any of the methods above which interfere with sperm manufacture. The treatment should affect within a few days only those sperm which are just ready for ejaculation. And when the drug is stopped, once any (perhaps damaged) sperm have been flushed out, the ones arriving fresh from the production line should hopefully not have been affected by it.

One of the first drugs tested for this effect was called *alpha-chlorohydrin*. More recently, *derivatives of ordinary sugar*, modified and containing chlorine atoms, had seemed very promising. In animal experiments they interfered with the fertilizing ability of already manufactured sperm, and when the treatment was stopped the animals were fertile again within a week. None of the drugs so far discovered has been found to be safe enough to use in man as they are toxic to the bone marrow and nervous system. But the basic idea is sound, and non-toxic alternatives are being sought.

Another spin-off from this research is that these chemicals, and also gossypol derivatives, are showing promise as more effective vaginal spermicides than those at present available.

Sperm transport from the epididymis onwards (stage ♂3)

Transport through the vas (stage ♂3a)

Vasectomy deserves to be and is very popular. It is a minor operation, basically a 'plumbing-job'. A small section of the vas is removed and the ends closed with catgut or by cautery (heat).

There are no proven serious long-term unwanted effects in men. It is true that in both men and animals, antibodies to sperm appear in quite a proportion. However, these are apparently not harmful in men; they do not even appear to interfere too much with the fertility of any individual after reversal of the operation. In spite of some reports in the medical journals and scare stories in the newspapers there is to date no agreement among the experts that these antibodies or any other effect of vasectomy can cause harm to the health of men after vasectomy. In this important respect men seem to be different from certain experimental animals.

Vasectomy taps and plugs

Vasectomy can be reversed, even when the original procedure was done by the usual methods. Using the operating microscope a team from St Louis in the United States are claiming the highest pregnancy rate quoted of 70 per cent. But the success rate 10 years after the original operation is much lower.

It is therefore attractive to consider devising some kind of *tap* which a man could turn on or off at will. Various such systems, one made of gold, have in fact been invented. They have not yet worked in practice because they were rejected by the tissues or became blocked. But even if taps were perfected, there is one snag which many people have not considered. Obviously turning the tap *on* should restore fertility almost at once. However, a man would have to wait perhaps up to three months after turning the tap off—just like after the original operation—before he could be sure that the downstream sperm had been flushed out and intercourse would not lead to a pregnancy. Ideally he should also get a pre-intercourse sperm count done. This is exactly the wrong way round, as many couples would happily wait three months to get their fertility back, but want their contraception to work straight away. However this would not be a serious objection to the tap approach (or more realistically a surgically removable plug, as reported recently from China), if it were only likely to be turned on/off once in the future, if at all.

Transport through the male urethra (stage ♂3b)

The mythical intra-penile device would work at this point. So, obviously, does the *sheath (condom)*. Research is going on into new designs including loose-fitting well-lubricated versions as part of the vital hunt for greater acceptability of this literally life-saving contraceptive method.

Immune methods

Research is going on in men, as in women, but so far progress has been disappointingly slow here as well.

The fact is that the practical male methods available now, or likely to appear in the forseeable future, remain, apart from withdrawal, simply the sheath and vasectomy. This is regrettable as women would very reasonably like men to take their share in this matter of birth control, and many men would like to be able to do just that. As making love itself is very much a sharing business, we badly need an adequately safe reversible hormonal method for each sex—so that each of a couple could take turns at being responsible for contraception. Each would then be exposed to half of any long-term risks of the methods.

Conclusion

This chapter could do no more than give a few examples, but at least it has given you a general framework for understanding future advances in family planning. Any future method you hear about has to be based on detecting or interfering with one of the stages in Figure 23.

Secondly, if you read reports of new methods, always be sceptical. Far too little money and scientific attention is directed to contraceptive research. In many countries drug regulatory committees have been created. They aim to ensure that new medicines and techniques are as safe as can be. But in the contraceptive drug field their understandable caution plus ever more litigation have had the effect of making development of new methods so expensive and prolonged (15 years is the minimum) as to tend to stop it altogether. Journalists often suggest that a brand-new method is just around the corner, when in fact it could be early next century before it is cleared for general use, if then. This can be irritating to many who find all the available methods unsatisfactory for one reason or another.

Thirdly, many women feel that they were betrayed during the 1960s over the problems of the original combined pill. Doctors are accused, not always fairly, of doing too little to warn users that there could be long-term problems. It seemed at that time a magical method, a panacea, 'the pill of the Brave New World'. Time has shown up its drawbacks, but these too have often been exaggerated. These lessons must be learned and applied when any new pill comes along, whether for use by men or by women.

Yet, for obvious reasons, the best of any future methods which may be devised will be those which act at just one stage in the reproductive process, and do not have any effects on the whole body at all—apart from good ones perhaps! And except in totally loyal relationships one of the latter will need to be a protective effect against sexually transmitted viruses.

10

....

All things considered: shall I take the pill?

The final decision has to be your own: books and doctors can only answer your questions, so far as the facts are known, and maybe give you some unbiased advice. But it is up to you to weigh up all the pros and cons, in consultation with your partner, and decide which method will suit you both best.

Your own 'best' method will depend on many things, among them: how crucial it is that you do not get pregnant; how much medical risk you feel prepared to accept; and how the actual method fits in with your sex life. Table 14 summarizes most of the pros and cons of the main recommended effective methods of birth control which are widely available, and may help you to make up your mind. Other methods which are *not* in the Table are missed out for the good reason that in the experience of most of the people who use them, they have a high failure rate.

No variety of *spermicide* is recommended for use on its own by normally fertile couples, even though in some countries spermicides are heavily promoted by manufacturers who imply that they are much more effective than they are. They appear in many different guises: pessaries, foaming tablets, creams, gels, ovals, films, and foams, also the *contraceptive sponge*, which is primarily a carrier for the contained spermicide. The sponge's failure rate in our Margaret Pyke Centre study was 24 per 100 woman-years, far too high for most young people to rely on. I recommend it because of its great acceptability in use for those who are 'spacing' and would accept an unplanned conception. It is otherwise useful as an *extra method* when fertility is already low for some reason: e.g. during breast-feeding; amenorrhoea (page 181); in the early months after the menopause, or above

Table 14 The main recommended and widely available methods of birth control

A. Reversible methods

Advantages	Disadvantages

The ordinary combined oral contraceptive (COC) pill

Advantages	Disadvantages
1. Extremely effective against pregnancy. Pregnancy rate in the range 0.2 to 1 per 100 woman-years.	1. Medical supervision required.
2. Independent of intercourse.	2. Needs a reasonably good memory to take the pills regularly.
3. Beneficial effects, especially on diseases connected with the menstrual cycle. See page 158.	3. Minor problems such as weight gain (page 159).
	4. A slight chance of major problems such as thrombosis.
	5. Especially unsuitable for women aged over 30–35 who are also heavy smokers.
	6. Some of the possible long-term consequences are still unknown.

The progestogen-only pill (mini-pill): see Chapter 8

Advantages	Disadvantages
1. Effective against pregnancy. Pregnancy rate 0.3 to 5 per 100 woman-years, the lower figure applying to older women.	1. Medical supervision required.
2. Independent of intercourse.	2. Needs to be taken obsessionally regularly.
3. Probably medically safer than the combined pill, as much less hormone is taken.	3. Minor problems, especially with the menstrual cycle.
4. Can be used by smokers aged over 35 and others for whom the combined pill is not recommended, or is proving unsatisfactory.	4. Very slight chance of major problems including ectopic pregnancy.
	5. Some of the possible long-term consequences still unknown.

Injectable (usually DMPA, Depo-Provera—see page 255)

Advantages	Disadvantages
1. Extremely effective against pregnancy. Pregnancy rate 0 to 1 per 100 woman-years.	1. Medical supervision required.
2. Independent of intercourse.	2. Disrupts the menstrual cycle, causing irregular bleeding or stopping the periods.
3. Beneficial effects: mostly as combined pill, including protection against pelvic infection.	3. *The injection cannot be removed* once given, so side-effects may have to be lived with for a long time.
4. Especially good for sickle cell anaemia.	4. Delay in return of fertility, though no permanent impairment.
5. Probably medically safer than the COC. Oestrogen free.	5. Minor problems such as weight gain.
	6. Some of possible long-term consequences unknown.

A. Reversible methods

Advantages	Disadvantages

IUD (loop or coil which is inserted into the uterus)

1. Effective against pregnancy. Pregnancy rate 0.3 to 4 per 100 woman-years, the lower figure applying to older women.
2. Independent of intercourse.
3. Nothing to remember: nothing to take or use daily.
4. No systemic effects, on the whole body.
5. Overall risk of death the same as or less than if the combined pill is used and, unlike it, becomes medically safer the older the user becomes.

1. Medical supervision required.
2. Insertion: can cause discomfort, and there is a very slight chance of perforation of the uterus.
3. The device may get expelled from the uterus into the vagina. This has to be watched out for.
4. May cause cramps, and heavy or prolonged or unpredictable bleeding.
5. Has certain medical risks, among them pelvic infection, miscarriage, and ectopic pregnancy. Pelvic infection is *rare*, *except* in IUD-users risking STDs (page 23).
6. Because the problems mentioned at 5 can lead to damage to one or both of the uterine tubes and hence interfere with future fertility, *not* an ideal method for women who have not yet had their family. Particularly unsuitable for most women under the age of 20. (DMPA may be a much better choice.)

The sheath or condom (preferably used with a spermicidal pessary, or lubricated with a spermicide)

1. Effective if used with care. Pregnancy rate 2 to 15 per 100 woman-years, can be as low as the IUD but very much depends on the user.
2. Easy to obtain at odd hours.
3. Good for infrequent intercourse.
4. May help a man who tends to climax too soon.
5. Visual proof that it has 'worked'.
6. NO MEDICAL RISKS WHATEVER.
7. No medical supervision required.
8. Protects against picking up or passing on sexually transmitted diseases, including viruses like that causing AIDS (i.e. safer sex, if not completely safe).

1. Needs very careful and consistent use.
2. Forward planning necessary, to have the sheath available every time.
3. Not independent of intercourse. Seems a 'messy' intrusion into love-making for some.
4. Both partners may be aware that it is being used. Loss of sensitivity much less with the newest designs which are spermicidally lubricated.
5. Can slip off or rupture in use.

A. Reversible methods

Advantages	Disadvantages

The cap which *must* be used with a spermicide (e.g. the diaphragm, which is put in by the woman to cover the entrance to the uterus)

Advantages	Disadvantages
1. Effective if used with care. Pregnancy rate 2 to 15 per 100 woman-years, can be as low as the IUD but very much depends on the user.	1. Medical supervision required, to choose the right size of cap and to be trained to use it properly.
2. More independent of intercourse than the sheath. Can be put in as a routine ahead of time and should not therefore interfere with spontaneity.	2. Needs very careful and consistent use.
3. Neither partner usually notices any loss of sensitivity.	3. Forward planning necessary.
4. If properly fitted and used, virtually no side-effects.	4. Seems a bit messy to some.
5. Protects against some sexually transmitted diseases.	5. Diaphragm may increase the risk of bladder infections. Other types of cap may be preferable if this is a problem.

B. Methods which are not readily reversible—sterilization in either sex

Advantages	Disadvantages

General pros and cons of sterilization in either sex

Advantages	Disadvantages
1. Almost but *not quite* 100 per cent effective.	1. Not readily reversible—but pregnancy rates after reversal operations by experts can be better than 50 per cent.
2. Independent of intercourse.	
3. Nothing to be taken daily.	2. An operation is required with more or less discomfort and inconvenience.
4. Medical supervision and possible problems mainly during the year of operation.	
5. No known long-term medical effects of importance, in the human.	

Pros and cons of female sterilization by blocking the uterine tubes

Advantages	Disadvantages
1. Once a woman decides to be sterilized, she is less likely in later years to want it reversed than a man might be, because nature will sterilize her anyway around the age of 50 (the menopause).	1. Medical risks of the operation are greater than vasectomy, though still small. Latest techniques using clips or rings are much safer than before.
2. The operation is immediately effective.	2. Usually requires admission to hospital and often (*not always*) a general anaesthetic.
	3. If the operation fails, which it very rarely does, there is a risk of ectopic pregnancy.

Advantages	Disadvantages
	4. Psychologically, though illogically, women may feel no longer so feminine because they cannot have babies.

Pros and cons of vasectomy (male sterilization) by blocking the vas deferens

1. Almost completely safe medically.	1. Occasional short-term local complications of the operation, such as swellings or infection.
2. Can be done under local anaesthetic, as an out-patient, almost anywhere.	2. The operation takes three or more months to become effective.
3. There is a ready check of success by doing sperm counts.	3. Especially if they re-marry, more older men than women will wish for a reversal operation (see the point about the menopause, above).
	4. Psychologically, though illogically, some men may feel 'threatened' by the operation, and may seem to overcompensate needlessly to show how manly they still are.
	5. Some *remotely* possible long-term effects still unknown, but most human evidence is reassuring (page 247).

age 50 anyway; or as a 'fail-safe' during use of another method like the IUD.

Of course sponges are a great deal better than nothing and the same applies to the *withdrawal method*, which some couples have used successfully for many years. (Its effectiveness can be improved by using a spermicidal foam or sponge *as well*.) Even if it works that one does tend to be rather frustrating. So are the present ovulation or '*natural methods*'; but future developments may give reliability with less abstinence (pages 240–1).

An advantage of the sheath and cap (and sponge) is that they only need to be used when necessary. There is none of the feeling that some women get when taking pills, for instance, that most of them are unnecessary since intercourse is so infrequent.

A note about the so-called 'messiness' of barrier methods of family planning such as *the sheath and the cap with spermicide*. This has been much exaggerated. And even if partly true, it is worth pondering the following comment which was made by a woman journalist: '. . . But women's lives are messy; it is messy to bleed once a month; it is messy to give birth; sex itself is not for the fastidious.'

A word about injectables: Depo-Provera (Table 14)

This is a progestogen injection called depot medroxyprogesterone acetate (DMPA for short), given into a muscle once every 12 weeks. It is brilliantly effective, with a failure rate in practice lower even than the COC because there are no tablets to forget. It seems very safe medically with so far no deaths proven to be caused by it. That clearly means it is even safer than the COC, without suggesting it is risk free.

Experiments showing that beagle dogs develop breast cancers probably have no relevance to humans since the beagle bitch has a high tendency to develop breast tumours, even under the influence of natural progesterone. There is some concern from New Zealand about long-term use of DMPA by young women, but at present most experts do not consider it increases the risk of human breast cancer.

DMPA has been very controversial, with accusations that it has been used in a racist way; also that women have received it without adequate counselling about its known or possible unknown risks. Wherever that has been true, that is an indictment of the doctors or other providers concerned, not of the drug. In the UK the licence as a contraceptive requires you to receive counselling aided by a special manufacturers' leaflet, which you should ask for if it is not offered.

Though still not approved for long-term contraceptive use in the USA, about 100 other countries including the UK permit its use, in some on a large scale. It has been 'tried and found *wanted*' by millions of women. The main point about Depo-Provera is that it is a first faltering step along a road which both the consumers and the providers of family planning would find very acceptable. It has disadvantages but these are well balanced by its advantages (Table 14). The alternative choice is Noristerat (also known as Norigest or Nur-Isterate), an oily injection of a norethisterone ester given every eight weeks.

How to plan your family planning

Some people will use only one or two methods of family planning throughout their lives; others will 'ring the changes' between the various methods shown in Table 14; for some a method such as the pill may be out of the question because of a medical contra-indication. But one thing is clear: whatever else applies, the best choice of method is likely to vary with time, or according to what I call in Table 15 'The seven contraceptive ages of woman'. But I do emphasize that Table 15 is just a guide: the choice of method of contraception is a very individual thing and no one method is ever ideal and best for everyone, even within a particular one of the seven categories. Not all the satisfactory options are even mentioned. The scheme only represents the 'state of the art' based on the methods available in the early 1990s. If some of the ideas in Chapter 9 become practical possibilities, then the ideal system might very well change.

Table 15 represents an ideal scheme, so it is assumed that the woman concerned will be a non-smoker and will, if she can, breast-feed her children. It is also assumed that she or her partner will use whatever method is chosen responsibly and consistently.

A main point to notice in the Table is that the pill is often the ideal method early on in fertile life, and if used at all the other main reversible 'medical' method of family planning, the IUD, is best reserved until later. This is because the known medical risks of the pill are less when you are young, and the younger you are the more secure you usually want to be against pregnancy. Besides, the 'fringe-benefits' like shorter and less painful periods are particularly appreciated. On the other hand, the IUD is relatively bad news for young women who have not yet completed their families, as it can be linked with various

Table 15 The seven contraceptive ages of woman

'Age'	Suggested method
1. Birth to puberty	No method required. However, responsible matter-of-fact sex education is essential—principally from the parents.
2. Puberty to marriage	Either (a) a barrier method (*sheath* or *cap* plus spermicide), or (b) the *combined pill / DMPA*, or (c) the 'best' oral contraceptive (i.e. saying 'no'). Choice depends on factors like religious views, the steadiness of the relationship, and frequency of intercourse.
3. Marriage to first child	First choice usually the *combined pill*, followed by a *barrier method* for three months before 'trying' for the first child.
4. During breast-feeding	First choice: *barrier method* (perhaps the *sponge*, or else either the *cap* or the *sheath*). Second choice: (a) *IUD* (but a small risk to future fertility, (b) the *POP* (but unknown effect of the minute amount of hormone transferred in the breast milk).
5. Family spacing after breast-feeding	Continue with method started during 4, or shift to *combined pill* at this time for greater effectiveness and a regular bleeding pattern.
6. After the (probable) last child	First choice: *IUD*. Other possibles: *barrier methods* or the *POP*, or continue *COC*, or *DMPA*, according to choice.
7. Family complete, children growing up and other methods unacceptable	*Vasectomy*; or *female sterilization* using clips or rings.

complications which could prejudice the chance of having a baby later—especially pelvic infection (infection of the uterine tubes) and ectopic pregnancy. However, by the sixth age in the Table, when your family is probably complete, but you are not yet quite ready for sterilization, those worries about the IUD are much less important. In addition most of the problems of the coil are less frequent in older women anyway. Moreover, unplanned pregnancy due to the device failing is definitely less likely in older women, particularly using the newest copper-band-carrying devices whose failure rate is as low as that of the pill! So the coil really comes into its own at the very time it is likely to be needed as an alternative, as the risks of the pill are increased in older women, especially smokers. The IUD can be a very useful 'holding manoeuvre' before your husband has his vasectomy (or you your sterilization).

Sterilization of either partner is often the ideal once the family is complete, because it is so safe medically and so effective against unplanned 'afterthoughts'. If you do not smoke, often it may be reasonable to take the slightly increasing medical risks with age of staying on the combined pill right through until either you or your partner is sterilized. However, it is not intended to imply that *everyone* should finish up by being sterilized. Indeed, it is important to remember about *female* sterilization that its risks become relatively more important after a woman passes 40, because there are then fewer years left in which to get the benefit from it before she reaches the menopause. Of course, how long this will be cannot be estimated in advance at all accurately. All that can be done is to balance the likely number of years of protection provided by the sterilization against the risks that are run during the actual year the operation is done. In developed countries the average age of the menopause is about 50.

Apart from sterilization, what methods are suitable for people during the seventh age, from the time when they are sure that their family is complete through until the time of the menopause? By the time they reach their forties a sizeable minority of around 10 per cent of women in Britain, and up to three times that number in some countries, have had their uterus removed (hysterectomy) for problems such as very heavy bleeding. Hysterectomy is of course a method of sterilization. But it is too big a procedure to be done routinely for family planning purposes. When it is medically indicated, good counselling is vital, as for other forms of sterilization.

In fact, many couples manage perfectly well using reversible methods of family planning right through to the menopause. Since the statement by that Committee of the US FDA many will now choose to stay on the appropriate combined pill (pages 105, 150). Many women find the IUD or the progestogen-only pill entirely satisfactory (but see pages 221–2). If they get irregular bleeding they should see their doctor to be sure it does not have a gynaecological explanation, before they assume it is due to their method. A surprisingly large number of people simply use the sheath or the cap at this time. Whatever reversible method is used, it should not normally be abandoned until one year after the very last menstrual period, as pregnancy during this time is not entirely unknown following an unexpected delayed egg-release. (But a blood test of the FSH level may speed the diagnosis of the menopause—see page 221.)

Combinations of methods

Some people really have difficulty in finding any method at all that suits them. Contraception can then be the source of a lot of tension and frustration. Occasionally a workable solution may be found if the partners, so to speak, share the contraceptive load: for instance, sometimes using the sheath and sometimes the diaphragm plus spermicide.

Using combinations of methods in a different way can help people who are terrified that a method will let them down. For example, the IUD can (very rarely) fail: especially in younger women under 30. If, however, they make a point of inserting a spermicidal pessary regularly every time before love-making, the effectiveness of their method can be improved.

Conclusion

Looking back over this chapter, and over the whole book, it is impossible to avoid one conclusion. A lot of the time in family planning we, and for the most part unfortunately that means women, are having to 'make the best of a bad job'. While we can hope for a successful outcome to some of the research described in Chapter 9, we have to *lead our sex lives now, with the methods actually available now.*

If you do decide to take the pill, and currently this is the most effective reversible method, make sure it is an informed decision which seems right to you and is not influenced by pressure from anyone else: your partner, the media, let alone any doctor. If you decide the pill is not for you, be sure to use some reliable alternative. Sex and birth control are matters which affect your body; they are your responsibility and require your decisions. That sums up the purpose for which this book was written.

100 questions everyone asks about the pill

Introduction

The answers to the questions here are deliberately very brief and hence sometimes over-simplified. Please refer to the pages mentioned for more details.

The two main types of pill are: POP = progestogen-only pill, COC = combined oral contraceptive pill. As in the rest of this book, the COC is often just called the pill, and because it is much more widely used than the POP, most of the questions and answers below refer to it.

(a) Types of pill and how they work

1. *What is the combined oral contraceptive pill (COC)?*
   This contains an oestrogen and progestogen and is usually taken daily, for 21 days out of every 28.
2. *How does it work?*
   Chiefly by stopping maturing and release of eggs (Chapter 2).
3. *What is the mini-pill/progestogen-only pill (POP)?*
   As its name suggests, this contains only a progestogen in very low dose, and is taken every single day of the year without breaks (Chapter 8).
4. *How does the POP work?*
   Chiefly by altering the cervical mucus to stop sperm entering the uterus, and by various changes to the lining of the uterus. See Chapter 8 for more details about this and other aspects of the POP.

5. *How effective are pills against pregnancy?*

   Very, if regularly taken. The failure rate of the COC is 0.2 to 1.0 pregnancies per 100 woman-years (page 47). The figure for the POP is 0.3 to 5 per 100 woman-years (page 209).

6. *Are all the combined pills the same?*

   No, there are differences between the brands, but we do not know which is the 'best buy' (pages 153–6). It seems best to take the lowest possible dose/body impact of both hormones: hence ultra-low-dose pills and POPs (Table 12, page 221) are preferred. But every woman is different, and some need the slightly higher-dose pills of Table 10 (page 188).

7. *What about phasic pills?*

   These are COCs giving a daily dose of both progestogen and oestrogen, but the ratio of one hormone to the other varies stepwise (see pages 192–5 for details). They may be either biphasic (two phases) or triphasic (three phases). Those available in Britain are ultra-low dose, but this is not necessarily true everywhere (see pages 301–5).

8. *How long has the pill been available?*

   The initial trials were in America and Puerto Rico in 1956. It was first marketed in the US in 1960, reaching most other countries in the early 1960s.

(b) Availability of the pill

9. *How can I get a supply of the pill?*

   In Britain over 90 per cent of family doctors will prescribe the pill. If your doctor will not, you should be able to obtain it from another local doctor, even if he or she is in a different practice; or from a Family Planning Clinic (addresses in the telephone directory).

10. *But I am under the age of consent . . . Will they insist on telling my parents?*

    These questions are answered on pages 82–4. If question 10 applies to you, the short sections on pages 23–8 and pages 28–31 might also be worth reading.

11. *Can my partner come to the clinic or surgery with me?*

Certainly and, if you ask, he can usually also come in with you when you see the doctor.

12. *Do I have to be examined internally at the first visit?*
No. The internal examination is primarily to do with preventive medicine. See pages 81–2. Once you are a pill-taker, regular checks of blood pressure and of headache pattern, breast examinations, and cervical smears are important (page 185).

13. *How often should I have a smear test done?*
This depends: policy varies from one district to another, so follow the advice of your doctor. An important factor is your own life-style (page 28), which could mean the need for annual testing whatever the local policy.

14. *They have asked me to come back for a smear test in only three months: what does this mean? Can I continue on the pill?*
No reason to panic: all this means is that a few abnormal cells have been found in the previous smear. Quite often these are got rid of by the body without any further treatment, and so are not seen on the repeat smear. Otherwise the doctor will discuss the whole matter with you. He or she will explain that even persistent changes in the smear can be readily dealt with and actual cancer of the cervix—which in any case would not occur for many years—can be prevented altogether by minor treatment, usually as an out-patient. See pages 28 and 81. And you should continue on the pill at least until you see your doctor, and possibly much longer—discuss in the light of pages 142–3, 184.

15. *How often should I attend the clinic or surgery for my pills?*
This will usually be determined by the number of packets you are given at each visit. Commonly you will be seen three months after first starting on the pill, and then regularly every six months. However, you must feel free to come back sooner than your next routine visit if you ever have any anxiety about using the pill or about any effect it seems to be having on you. See also Question 20 below about special medical supervision.

(c) Practical pill-taking

16. *Which diseases that I have ever suffered from should I be sure to mention to the doctor?*

    The main thing to mention is any past thrombosis or any disease or disorder affecting the circulation (pages 171–3). These include diabetes, high blood pressure, and heavy cigarette-smoking. Liver troubles should be mentioned; the other important short- and long-term disorders are to be found on pages 171–84. Allergies, especially to drugs, should also be entered in your case notes.

17. *What diseases in my family are important?*

    Once again, any history of thrombosis or any kind of stroke is important, but only if it affected a near-relative at a young age (say under 50). Mention also if there is a family tendency to breast cancer, or raised blood pressure or diabetes (pages 141, 178). When in doubt mention any unusual family complaint, especially porphyria (page 175) and otosclerosis (page 176).

18. *Who should never take the pill?*

    Having noted the diseases in your own past or still affecting you, or those which run in your family, the final decision about this will be taken by your doctor in consultation with you. See pages 171–85.

19. *Who should be very cautious about taking the pill and then only with special medical supervision?*

    Again, this will depend on your own medical history and that of your family (pages 177–84). If one of these 'relative contra-indications' applies, it is usually essential to use a COC giving the minimum possible dose with the selected progestogen—or the POP (page 221).

20. *What does 'special medical supervision' mean?*

    It means (pages 184–5) being seen by the doctor more often than usual, being told what to look out for so as to return earlier if necessary, and sometimes having special tests done. It also means being ready to discontinue the pill should some condition worsen, or a new risk factor or problem appear.

21. *There seems to be no medical objection, so how do I start taking the pill?*

There are two main ways, but you should usually start with the first tablet on day 1 of the period (pages 54–5 and Figure 10). The POP should always be started on day 1 (page 210). See also pages 55, 210 for how to start COCs and POPs after any kind of recent pregnancy.

22. *Which pill is best if I plan to breast-feed my baby?*

The POP—but first read carefully the discussion on pages 222–3.

23. *How soon after starting the pill am I protected against pregnancy?*

At once, if either the COC or POP are started early enough after a full-term baby; or if either is started by the day after a miscarriage or termination of pregnancy, or on day 1 of the menstrual cycle—or even by day 4 (see post-coital contraception, pages 78–9). Otherwise alternative precautions such as the sheath should be used until seven tablets have been taken (page 54).

24. *How do I take the pills after that?*

You take 21 consecutive daily pills followed by a 7-day break for all the available COCs (pages 186–9). Every Day pills contain dummies to be taken during the pill-free week. Like them, the POP is taken every single day including during periods. With *all* pills tablet-taking should continue following the daily routine, even if there is unexpected bleeding (pages 72 and 209 and Question 51 below).

25. *Is it safe to make love on the days when COCs are not taken?*

Yes: *but only* if no pills have been missed (or not absorbed) towards the end of the previous pill packet, and you do in fact start another packet after the pill-free week (pages 53–4).

26. *Do I have to take pills at the same time of day, and if so what time is best?*

For COCs, any regular time will do. POPs should be taken within an hour of the same time each day. For many the best time is in the early evening. The worst time for this pill is just before the usual time for love-making (page 210).

27. *How can I ever remember to take my pills?*
Some women find it helpful to take one of the Every Day packs of COCs, which contain 21 active tablets and seven dummies so there is no need to remember when to stop and start successive courses. Get your pill-taking routine linked with something else that you do regularly every day. For instance, you could tie your packet of COCs to your tooth-brush. An alarm watch set to 7 o'clock in the evening, or any meal-time, may be safest for the POP.

28. *I have forgotten to take a pill: am I likely to get pregnant?*
No, especially if you are on the COC, and with both types of pill if you do not rely on pills for the recommended time (see Question 29).

29. *What shall I do?*
COCs: if more than 12 hours late in pill-taking, take one missing pill and then continue in all respects as usual with your pill-taking routine, but use the sheath or a similar method for the next seven days. *If and only if* you find you have missed one or more of the last seven tablets in the packet, throw out the rest! Start with pill number one of a new pack *at once*, missing out any 'reminder tablets'. See Figure 11 and pages 58–65 for further details. If it was a missed POP extra precautions must be used for 48 hours even if you were only 3 hours late in taking a tablet (see Figure 21, pages 212–13, and the Important Note on page 211).

30. *What shall I do if I have a stomach upset—vomiting or diarrhoea?*
As far as your body is concerned, this can be like missing a tablet. See Figures 12 or 21 (pages 67–8, 212–13) for the rules to be followed with COCs or POPs for maximum peace of mind.

31. *Can other medicines affect the reliability of the COCs and POPs?*
Yes, some can. This particularly applies to some antibiotics and to treatments for tuberculosis and for epilepsy. Bleeding on COC-taking days may be an early

warning sign (Table 3 and pages 67–72, 214).

32. *Can the pill affect the actions of other medicines?*
Again, this is possible, depending on the nature of the other treatment. See page 72, for COCs; there are no reports of this with POPs.

33. *Should I then always make a special point of telling any doctor who sees me that I am on the pill?*
Yes. This is vital, not only because of this problem of interaction between drugs, but also because laboratory tests may be affected (page 87); and the knowledge that you are on the COC or POP may also help when making a diagnosis or planning surgery.

34. *Does it matter if I accidentally take more than one pill per day?*
No. In fact this is sometimes recommended (Figure 11b, page 61). However, if you make this mistake, it is best to take your *next* pill from another packet, so that the day of pill-taking matches the day marked on your current one.

35. *If a change to a different brand of COC is recommended, are there any special rules?*
Yes. If moving to a pill on the same 'rung' of Figure 17 (pages 190–1), or higher, just take the usual 7-day break between old and new packets. But if moving *down* to a lower-dose pill or if in doubt, take the first new packet without any break after the old one (page 72). See page 193 for the rules for phasic pills, and page 211 if moving to the POP, or from the POP to any other method.

36. *If I lose my COCs half-way through a packet and my friend has a spare packet of a different brand, is it safe to take them?*
Forget this if either yours or hers are phasic pills (page 192). Even if they are of the fixed-dose type, it is *not* recommended. However, if there seems no alternative, perhaps when you are away for a weekend, then you should certainly check that the pill is on an equivalent rung of the ladders of Figure 17. If it is higher, protection will be maintained, but if lower, then it may be reduced and you should preferably follow the 7-day loss-of-protection rule, as well as taking the new pills. (The same

rule, or running on the packets as on page 72, is best followed when you return to your normal pill from a borrowed higher-dose one!)

37. *What shall I do if I need some more pills when in a foreign country?*
Look up your variety of pill in the World directory of pill names (page 301). You should then be able to use the name of the nearest equivalent locally available brand when you visit the doctor or chemist.

38. *If my partner goes abroad, or I get a side-effect, can I stop the pill in the middle of a packet?*
With the COC it is best to complete the packet. But if you have one of the possibly serious symptoms mentioned on page 75, you should still be able to avoid a pregnancy if you transfer immediately to using another method like the sheath. POPs are best stopped during a period (page 211) so this could be before the end of a packet.

39. *Does it matter if I take the pill for short spells of a few months at a time, according to need?*
No, so long as the rules for starting and stopping are followed each time (see Questions 23, 25, and 38).

40. *If I want a baby, can I just stop the pill? Or should I use another method for a while?*
See pages 128–30 for the answer to this one and to Question 77 (about pill-taking *during* pregnancy). It seems that previous use of the pill does not increase the chance of having an abnormal baby.

41. *What should I do if I am not quite sure whether I have had German measles? Or whether I was vaccinated against it as a schoolgirl?*
German measles in early pregnancy can harm babies, so you should not stop the pill until you have had the blood test to check that you are immune (pages 81–2).

42. *If I am not immune, how long must I wait after the vaccination for German measles before getting pregnant?*
One month is now advised (page 82). So it is logical to get this matter sorted out while you are still taking the COC or POP, or using some other effective method.

43. *I am going into hospital for an operation—should I stop*

the pill and if so, when? And when can I take it again?

Much depends on whether this is for a major or a minor operation. If you are told you will be in hospital for several days after the operation, then you should transfer from the COC to another effective method four weeks beforehand. There is normally no need to discontinue the POP in this way, but discuss the matter with your doctor. If there are no complications you can restart the pill *at the first subsequent period which comes on at least two weeks following full mobility after the operation.* See pages 174–5.

44. *Does being sterilized count as a major operation?*

Not if done by modern laparoscopy techniques. Therefore there is no need to stop the COC, and usually it is best to continue pill-taking after the operation until the end of the current packet.

45. *How long can I stay on the pill? Should I make a break every two years? Or after five years?*

The effect of the length of pill-use on the risks of diseases of the circulation and cancer has not yet been fully worked out (pages 149–52). But it is clear that the uncommon infertility problem of amenorrhoea—absent periods for many months—after stopping the pill is no more likely after long-term than short-term use. So it is not necessary, as used to be recommended, to make a routine break every two years.

According to present knowledge and depending on other factors which apply to you, it is preferable after 10–15 years' use of the COC *to begin to consider whether to move to another method.* However it could be OK for you to use it much longer if you are a healthy non-smoker (pages 149–52). (The risks, if any, of long-term use of the POP are thought to be even less than those of the COC.)

(d) Pills and periods, or no periods

Combined oral contraceptive pill (COC)

46. *What causes 'periods' on the COC? Are they really periods at all?*

    The natural menstrual cycle is abolished whether or not you see any bleeding. It is replaced by the pill cycle in which bleeding is caused in a quite different way, by withdrawal of the hormones from the blood supply to the uterus for seven days out of every 28. So they are not true periods (page 47 and Figure 9).

47. *I have irregular periods naturally—can I take the pill?*

    This depends: special tests may be required. An important factor is whether you would accept an alternative (not the IUD). See pages 126 and 181.

48. *I have missed a 'period'—what shall I do?*

    If you have no reason to suspect loss of protection by the pill (pages 58–72), you should start a new packet after the pill-free week in the usual way. However, if the next pill withdrawal bleed also fails to come—i.e. you miss two 'periods' in a row—you should see your doctor before starting another packet (page 65).

49. *If I don't see much of a 'period'/I see no bleeding at all in the pill-free week, is blood collecting inside me?*

    No—as explained on pages 47–9, if you have no bleeding it simply means there is no blood to come away. Check you are not pregnant, and then if you wish you can continue with the pill (Figure 20b, pages 200–2), if your doctor agrees.

50. *Can I avoid having monthly bleeding altogether—e.g. when going on holiday?*

    Yes: the best way is to take two packets in a row (page 53). But there are special rules for phasic pills (page 195).

51. *What is the tricycle pill?*

    This is the ordinary pill, but refers to a system of taking usually three packets in a row followed by a 7-day break pages 52–3). It gives only four to five hormone withdrawal bleeds a year, and has some important uses (pages 53, 182, 183). But it also means that, overall, more hormone is taken in the time. NB Do not confuse this with the triphasic pill—see Question 7.

52. *I am bleeding like a period on days of pill-taking: should I stop in the middle of a packet?*

On no account! The golden rule of pill-taking is to carry on taking your pills according to the 21 days on, 7 days off routine, irrespective of the pattern of bleeding or no-bleeding which may occur. See page 200 (Figure 20a) and make an early appointment to discuss this with your doctor, particularly if it is a new problem.

53. *I not only get spotting on pill-taking days, I have had no bleeding during the last seven days of no tablet-taking! What shall I do?*

Actually, this is quite a common combination of problems. If you have no reason to suspect loss of protection from the pill, and this is the first missed 'period', then follow the rules at Question 48 above and start taking your next packet on the correct day. If you persevere, taking your pills regularly, there is a good chance that the correct bleeding pattern will be established. If not, you should make an early appointment to discuss things with your doctor (Figure 20 and pages 200–2).

Irregular bleeding like this is even more likely to happen after erratic pill-taking, or some other reason for loss of protection (pages 58 72). If this applies to you, then follow the rules of Figures 11 or 12 and page 66, and take your doctor's advice before starting another packet.

Progestogen-only pill (POP)

54. *What causes periods on the POP?*

Quite unlike the COC, these periods are natural ones: due to the loss of the natural progesterone and oestrogen, as egg-release and formation of a corpus luteum often occur (page 208).

55. *Does it matter if I see no periods on the POP?*

Yes and no. First check you are not pregnant. If not, this means you are as protected against pregnancy as if you were on the COC (page 215). It may mean your natural menstrual cycle is particularly easy to stop; the POP should not be appreciably harming your fertility and can be continued. See pages 216–17 and discuss the matter with your doctor.

56. *What should I do if I get erratic bleeding and spotting on the POP?*
Continue daily pill-taking: if the bleeding pattern is unacceptable see your doctor.

Periods after stopping the pill—either the COC or POP

57. *Although I had very regular 'periods' on the pill I stopped it some months ago and have seen no periods yet. What does this mean?*
It means that your natural menstrual cycle, with egg-release and periods, has not yet been restored. It usually will be without treatment (pages 76–7, 126–7 and see Question 58).

58. *We have been trying to have a baby since stopping the pill with no success yet. Was the pill to blame and should we have tests done?*
Between 10 and 15 per cent of all couples have difficulty achieving a pregnancy, so it *could* be a coincidence. Discuss referral for tests with your doctor if you see no periods for six months or more, or you could wait a few months longer if periods have returned.

59. *Could using the pill for a long time make my menopause happen earlier? or later?*
Neither the COC nor POP are thought to have any effect on the time of the menopause.

60. *If I am on the POP, how do I find out that I have reached the menopause?*
The usual way is to transfer to another method. It may sometimes be possible to confirm the menopause by a blood test—discuss with your doctor and see page 221, also Question 76 below.

(e) Problems with the pill

61. *How dangerous, really, is the COC?*
    Like any drug it has risks, but these have often been exaggerated. One very good point is that no harm is likely to be caused by a large overdose (pages 85–6).

62. *How dangerous is the POP?*
    Probably even less so than the COC (page 217).

63. *What side-effects will I notice?*
    Often none at all. If you do, it is nearly always worth persevering (but see Question 64), at least for three months. Even then, do not give up the method too easily: there are other brands of COC or POP which might be tried.

64. *What symptoms should make me see a doctor at once?*
    These are listed on page 75, but they are very rare so do not let the list worry you!

65. *Won't I put on a lot of weight?*
    Usually none with the POP, and very little if any with the modern ultra-low-dose COCs. But you may need to count calories a little more carefully (page 92). If you are already overweight, see pages 172, 180.

66. *Could the pill be causing my headaches?*
    It is possible, especially if they happen on the pill-free days. This could be a good reason for tricycling, page 52. Bad headaches or migraines should always be discussed with your doctor (pages 111–12).

67. *I get so depressed these days: how likely is it that the pill is to blame?*
    There may sometimes be a clear-cut link with the pill (page 108), but often there is not. Vitamin B_6 may help.

68. *I seem to have lost interest in sex too; would stopping the pill help?*
    Not very often. Could there be something wrong within your sexual relationship? Transferring to an oestrogen-dominant pill or the POP is worth trying. If the problem is partly a feeling of vaginal dryness, a check-up for thrush (Candida) infection and/or using a jelly lubricant may also help (page 110).

69. *Could the brown blotches I have started to get on my face be due to the pill?*

    Yes they could, they are given the name chloasma (page 134). The POP may help, if you still want to take a pill.

70. *Since starting on the pill I feel sick and dizzy and have too much vaginal discharge—what shall I do?*

    All these may well improve after two or three courses of pills; nausea can often be reduced by taking the pills last thing at night. Otherwise these and other symptoms, which seem to be due to too much oestrogen effect in comparison with the progestogen effect, can be helped by using a progestogen-dominant pill, or by the progestogen-only pill (page 203).

71. *Thrombosis sounds very worrying: I am told it means clots, so does it mean that I can't use the pill if I have clots with my periods?*

    Far from it: clots with the periods just mean that they are heavy, and could well improve dramatically if you went on the pill (page 124).

72. *What are the facts about thrombosis and other troubles of the circulation?*

    Chapters 4 and 6 are mainly about this. In brief, the risk is primarily in people who have other risk factors, listed on pages 97–8. Smoking is the most common and main one, and becomes even more important as age increases (pages 105–6).

73. *Which reduces this risk more, to stop the pill or to stop smoking?*

    For anyone smoking 15 or more cigarettes a day, the risks of all the currently available pills are less overall than those of smoking. However long you have been a smoker, your chances of survival are always greater if you stop (page 107).

74. *I smoke 25 cigarettes a day: how can I be helped to stop?*

    In Britain, ASH (Action on Smoking and Health—see useful addresses, page 298) can give you practical advice and there may be an anti-smoking clinic you could attend. But there is no magic method: you will never succeed unless you really want to give up, and you are prepared to work hard to do so.

75. *At what age should I stop the pill?*

    There is no set age. The risk increases steadily with time; it depends on whether you have any other risk factors, and is thought not to apply much to the POP. See pages 105–7, 149–52, 180, 221, and discuss with your doctor.

76. *I am near the 'change of life', and I have been given treatment for hot flushes. The pills are in a packet which looks very like 'the Pill' and I take them just the same way. Are they contraceptives?*

    No! If you were still having periods up to the time of starting this treatment, which is known as 'hormone replacement therapy', you should not rely on it. The dose system is different, and may not be effective in preventing pregnancy. It could be more appropriate for you to switch to using the COC, especially Mercilon. See pages 105, 189–92.

77. *If I got pregnant and did not realize, would continuing to take the pill harm the baby?*

    The risk of this is very low indeed, if it exists, and did not show up among 168 babies (page 129).

78. *Does the evidence we have so far suggest that the overall risk of cancer is greater in pill-users than in those who never take the pill?*

    No: see pages 138–46.

79. *Have the risks of the pill sometimes been exaggerated?*

    Yes. Even more commonly, the problems of the pill are not put in perspective against its benefits, or in comparison with the risks and problems of alternatives, of using no method at all, and of life generally (pages 162–70).

80. *What about the risks for people in developing countries?*

    These are probably less than in 'over-developed' countries, also the risks of alternatives and of pregnancy tend to be greater there. But much more research is needed (pages 147–8).

81. *Are there still things we don't know about the pill, particularly about long-term risks?*

Yes (pages 149–56). This book can do no more than give a consensus or majority view on the known facts about the pill. Very preliminary findings are not mentioned, because it would be as wrong to cause false fears as it would be to raise false hopes.

82. *After all that, what good effects does the pill have?*
See Table 7 (pages 158–9). Main ones are that it is highly effective, acceptable, and unrelated to intercourse, and almost 100 per cent reversible; plus its good effects on two cancers and on the menstrual cycle in most women.

(f) People in special categories (if your situation is not mentioned here, please use the index)

83. *Does it affect my choice of pill that I am very underweight?*
Underweight women are more likely to have side-effects like menstrual cramps, nausea, and breast discomfort, and to have a long delay in return of their periods after stopping the pill. Hence they should be given either a combined pill with lowest possible dose, or the POP. See page 197.

84. *Can I take the combined pill if I have varicose veins?*
Yes, on their own these rarely mean that you must avoid the method. Please make a point of reading pages 95–6.

85. *Can I take the COC if I am a diabetic?*
Sometimes, but only if you do not smoke, have no diabetic complications, and with special medical supervision for the shortest possible time (pages 172, 178). The POP could be a better choice.

86. *I am very troubled by acne, does this affect which pill I should take?*
Yes it does: you should use a relatively oestrogen-dominant pill (page 204).

87. *Can I use contact lenses if I take the pill?*
Probably: with modern lenses and modern ultra-low-dose COCs (and POPs). But if your eyes ever become sore do not use the lenses until you have seen your optician again

for them to be examined, and for advice (page 114).

88. *I tend to be anaemic, can I take the pill?*
    It depends. If you have one of the commonest kinds of anaemia, due to heavy periods, the pill will be a great help (page 124). But if you have sickle cell anaemia (only possible if you have some negro blood in you) discuss the matter with your doctor (pages 179–80).

89. *Does the fact that I have recently had infectious hepatitis (jaundice) mean that I cannot ever again take the pill?*
    No, but it does mean that you must have blood tests done to check when your liver is functioning normally, and you will usually be advised to stay off both COC and POP for as long as you must avoid alcohol, normally at least three months (page 175).

90. *What about the very itchy mild jaundice that I had in pregnancy?*
    This, like other conditions which are definitely or probably affected by any type of sex hormones (page 117), means you should always avoid the pill.

91. *Does it matter that I had high blood pressure (toxaemia) in pregnancy?*
    This must be mentioned to your doctor, and your blood pressure will need to be checked more often than usual. But most women with this history do not have any trouble later on the pill *if they avoid smoking* (pages 97, 179).

92. *I had a funny kind of miscarriage, and am now having regular blood tests. What can this mean?*
    You presumably had trophoblastic disease—ask your doctor to confirm, and see page 144 for a full explanation. If so, you will have to avoid both the COC and POP, but only till you are given the 'all-clear' by your doctor, based on the hCG tests.

(g) Miscellaneous

93. *Should I avoid any foods or alcohol, or take extra vitamins while on the pill?*
    As a rule, no (pages 91–2). But see also pages 108–9, 128.

94. *I am going on a long scheduled flight to Australia. I am on the pill, are there any precautions I should take?*

Yes there are. As mentioned on page 174, high altitude increases the risk of thrombosis. Especially if you are a bit overweight and tend to be sedentary, even though the plane will be pressurized to about the equivalent of 2,000 metres, thrombosis in the leg veins is indeed more likely. There is no necessity to come off the pill—many flight attendants use it all the time. But follow their example and take some exercise during the flight: such as a brief walk around the plane every hour or so.

95. *What shall I do, my 3-year-old daughter has just swallowed all the pills in my next packet . . .?*

Nothing—provided you are sure that this is all she took. She may vomit, and within the next day or two she may have some painless bleeding from her uterus, like a light period. This sounds alarming but is actually no cause for concern (page 85).

96. *If the pill stops release of eggs, what happens to the eggs?*

They stay in the ovary, just as they would in a woman who was perpetually pregnant. However, there is always a steady loss of egg cells within the ovary, from before birth right through to the menopause (page 34).

97. *What is the injection/jab/jag/shot?*

These words and others are used to describe that most useful injectable contraceptive called DMPA or Depo-Provera, and various other progestogens which are being tried by this route (pages 229, 251, 255).

98. *What is the 'morning-after' pill? (a bad name, page 78).*

This describes methods which are used after intercourse to prevent pregnancy. A lot of research is being done, but the few methods available now are only suitable for 'emergency' use. See pages 78–9, 234.

99. *What about the male pill?*

I am sorry to say this is still very much in the future. There is no safe, acceptable pill for men now, nor is there likely to be one for several years to come (pages 242–7).

100. *What if I have any other questions about ANYTHING?*

Ask them and keep on asking them: pertinent or

impertinent questions! It is your body, and you have a right to know. Never hesitate to go back to whoever prescribed your pills to discuss all aspects of pill-taking. But remember that some facts simply are not yet available.

Postscript

As I said on page 30, I feel no doctor involved in family planning should push his or her own moral views on those who come for advice. They should be met on their own ground. In all but the most unusual case, if an unmarried couple are having intercourse frequently it would be alienating and probably quite useless to suggest that they abstain. Circumstances vary, but the main thing is to help people avoid the nightmare of an unwanted pregnancy. I feel it is not my role to judge, but to care. Although my own views often differ from the views of those to whom I prescribe the pill, to draw attention to this, except at their request, might mean losing the opportunity to help them (often not just with their contraception).

So I do prescribe the pill without moralizing to unmarried people: and also, with counselling, which is not the same as moralizing, to young teenagers. We live in the real world of the 1990s and my medical practice must be relevant to that world.

Though I must practise my profession in the real world this does not mean that I think all is well there in matters of sex and responsibility. Far from it. I am not in favour of the life-style that contributes to increasing numbers of broken marriages; single-parent families; induced abortions; not to mention prescriptions for tranquillizers for more and more insecure housewives and their partners, quite unable to trust each other. The 'copulation explosion' is the root cause of the epidemic of sexually transmitted diseases; and also, we now know, of abnormal cervical smears and the risk of cancer of the cervix. So I see it as sound medicine, not being 'holier than thou', to point out to a patient I have had to treat for pelvic infection due to a sexually transmitted disease that her future fertility could be damaged if she does not change her life-style; or to reinforce a teenager's wish, if she has it, *not* to be given the pill just yet, because she really does not feel ready for intercourse (or wishes to wait till she marries). Unfortunately, we live in a society which has rejected old values but can offer nothing satisfactory instead; a society where many young people receive little guidance, and plenty of bad examples. The pressures on them from the media and their friends are enormous, to the extent that it really seems to be abnormal not to be having sex at 16. Or, as a family doctor said, 'Sex at 16 may be legal but it is not yet compulsory!'

Concerned as they rightly are to prevent unplanned pregnancy, sometimes school teachers and doctors can be implicated in these social pressures. They can find that their promotion of family planning is being seen as implying an official seal of approval for teenage sex.

The young will laugh at an arbitrary 'not at all', but will at least listen to a case for 'not yet', if it is factual and not linked to taboos or a negative attitude to sex. They need to know that the price to be paid for sexual intercourse in their early teens *can* be too high. At risk are self-respect, respect for others, and emotional security: their own and that of their children in the future. These facts apply to boys as well as girls. The sexual 'double standard' is offensive and must be abolished! But for girls there are also relevant medical facts: all contraceptives *can* fail, and the possible long term risks may include infertility and even AIDS and cancer (see pages 25, 26 and 28.)

The stakes are also high for adults. In the book *I Married You* (Further reading, page 292), the author compares sexual love to glue between two pieces of paper. 'If you try to separate two pieces of paper which are glued together, you tear them both. If you try to separate husband and wife who cleave together, both are hurt—and in those cases where they have children, the children as well. Divorce means to take a saw and to saw apart each child, from head to toe, right through the middle.' The imagery is too vivid, perhaps, but it rings true.

Personally, I am now a convinced Christian. I believe that the sexual behaviour we were designed for can be summed up as 'A one-man woman who makes love only with her one-woman man . . . for life'. I can accept that some who consider this notion old fashioned, and reject it, are nevertheless responsible. They can perhaps avoid unwanted pregnancies and STDs and succeed in not hurting each other or third parties and, most importantly, can in due course bring their children up in secure homes based on mutual trust. But are not these good outcomes more *likely* down the other road?

There are many types and many different outlooks in this troubled world. This postscript was written so that you, reading this book, might know where I stand.

Glossary

abortion: loss of a pregnancy at any time before independent existence apart from the mother is deemed to be possible. Abortion may be *spontaneous* (= miscarriage) or *induced*, meaning caused to happen either legally or illegally. The general public often uses the word 'abortion' on its own to mean a legal induced abortion, but doctors prefer to use either that phrase or *termination of pregnancy.*

allergy: abnormal reactivity of an individual to a specific substance, following previous exposure to the same or a closely related substance. A similar process to *immunity* (below), but the *antibodies* produced are unwanted and can be harmful.

amine: an organic compound which contains nitrogen. The ones referred to in this book are present in the brain and believed to be important in its functions, both in health and disease.

anaemia: a decrease in the blood of the substance haemoglobin, carried by the red blood cells, which transports oxygen round the body.

androgenic: masculinizing.

antibodies: special substances produced by the body as a reaction to a foreign substance, or a substance which the body treats as foreign (page 237). Antibodies can be beneficial (as in *immunity*) or harmful (as in *allergy*).

'breakthrough' bleeding: any unexpected bleeding between hormone withdrawal bleeds ('periods') on the combined pill: i.e. bleeding on pill-taking days.

cervix: the narrow lower end of the *uterus*, containing the entrance to it. Sometimes called 'the neck of the womb'.

chlamydia: the commonest cause of sexually transmitted infection of the fallopian tubes, also known as salpingitis or pelvic infection, which can lead to sterility from blocked tubes.

chloasma (= melasma): abnormal facial skin pigmentation occurring in some women during pregnancy or oral contraception.

chromosome: one of the microscopic thread-like structures visible in the nucleus of any body cell when it divides, carrying the genes. (Each gene controls the inheritance of a special characteristic of the individual—e.g. blood group or colour of the eyes.)

combined oral contraceptive: contraceptive which is taken by mouth and contains two hormones: one a *progestogen* and the other an *oestrogen*.

cone biopsy: a minor operation to remove some skin at the entrance to the uterus in order to treat abnormal cells found by cervical smear.

contraception: prevention of pregnancy by a reversible method. This definition excludes the other two types of birth control, which are sterilization and abortion. But see pages 235–6.

contraceptive: any substance or device which produces contraception.

corpus luteum: the yellow body formed in the ovary during the menstrual cycle, arising from the largest follicle after it has discharged the egg.

cystitis: inflammation of the urinary bladder, usually caused by infection, causing a desire to pass urine more frequently and frequently a burning sensation on doing so.

D & C (Dilatation and Curettage): a very common minor operation in which the cervix is dilated, or enlarged sufficiently to allow a curette to be passed. This instrument is then used to scrape the lining of the inside of the uterus, in order to empty it, e.g. after a miscarriage or induced abortion which has been incomplete, or to obtain tissue for laboratory examination.

diabetes: strictly, should be *diabetes mellitus*—a disturbance of body chemistry causing an increase in the level of glucose in the blood after food, due to lack of the hormone insulin, or reduction in its effectiveness. These changes can lead to long-term complications, especially affecting the arteries.

ectopic pregnancy: a pregnancy in the wrong place—i.e. anywhere other than in the cavity of the uterus. The commonest site is in the uterine tube. It leads to the need for urgent operation, because the growing pregnancy can cause internal bleeding.

ejaculation: the spurting out of semen (sometimes called *the ejaculate*) from the end of the penis when a man has a climax.

embolism: transfer in the bloodstream of a mass, such as a blood clot from a vein, to lodge elsewhere, generally in the lungs (*pulmonary embolism*, page 94).

embryo: name given to the early pregnancy from conception until about two months (then called the fetus).

endometrium: the special lining of the uterus, which is prepared by the hormones of the menstrual cycle in readiness for implantation of an embryo—or otherwise is shed at the menstrual period.

enzyme: a biological catalyst, which is a chemical which promotes the process of transformation of one substance to another within the body.

epididymis: a long tube coiled on itself to form a small linear structure attached to the testicle, and connecting it with the vas deferens.

ethinyloestradiol: one of the two artificial oestrogens which are used in combined oral contraceptive pills.

fertilization: the union of sperm and egg cell. The fertilized egg divides and implants to produce an embryo and eventually a new individual.

fimbriae: the seaweed-like fronds which surround the outer end of each uterine tube, like a fringe.

follicle: a small fluid-filled balloon-like structure in the ovary, containing an egg cell. Only one, out of about 20 which enlarge in each menstrual cycle, normally releases a mature egg.

FSH (follicle stimulating hormone): the hormone produced by the pituitary gland which stimulates the growth of follicles in the ovary; and hence causes the production of oestrogen and the maturing of an egg cell in the largest follicle.

hCG (human chorionic gonadotrophin): the hormone, produced by an early pregnancy, which travels to the ovary in the bloodstream and causes its corpus luteum to continue producing oestrogen and progesterone beyond its usual 14-day life span. The action of hCG is hence very similar to that of LH (see below).

hormone: a chemical substance produced in one organ and carried in the bloodstream like a 'chemical messenger' to another organ or tissue, whose function it influences or alters.

hypertension: high blood pressure, above the level which is accepted as normal (pages 102–3).

hysterectomy: an operation to remove the uterus.

immunity: resistance of the body to the effects of a foreign substance, resulting from the production of *antibodies* (see above) which are not harmful and are often beneficial—unlike those produced as a result of *allergy.*

implantation: the process of embedding of the developing embryo in the endometrium.

IUD (intra-uterine device): a small plastic device, which may or may not also bear a chemical such as copper, which is inserted into the uterus to prevent pregnancy. Often called the 'coil' or 'loop'.

LH (luteinizing hormone): the hormone produced by the pituitary gland which causes egg-release, and the production and maintenance of the corpus luteum.

libido: the internal urge or drive associated with the sexual instinct.

lipids: fats and associated chemical substances, carried in the blood.

mcg (microgram): this abbreviation is used of the metric unit which is one-millionth of a gram in weight.

menopause: cessation of the menstrual periods due to failure of ovulation and hormone production by the ovaries. Often used inaccurately for the climacteric, the period of several years before and after periods actually cease.

menstrual cycle: the cycle of hormone and other changes in a woman's body which leads to a regular discharge of blood from the non-pregnant uterus.

mestranol: the less commonly used of the two artificial oestrogens in combined oral contraceptive pills.

mucus: slippery fluid produced by mucous glands on the surface of a body structure. *Cervical mucus* is mucus produced by the glands of the cervix.

oestrogen: the female sex hormone produced by the ovary throughout the menstrual cycle. It is the hormone required to bring animals 'on heat', which occurs at the time called oestrus—hence the name oestrogen.

oestrogen-dominant pill: a combined pill whose biological effects on the body are due more to the relatively higher dose of oestrogen it contains than to the progestogen.

ovary: the female sex gland in which ova (egg cells) are developed and which is the main source of natural sex hormones.

ovulation: discharge of the ovum from the ovary—usually called egg-release in this book.

phlebitis: thrombosis and inflammation involving a vein—usually a superficial vein of the leg—which causes it to become hard and very tender.

pituitary gland: the gland, about the size of a pea, on a stalk at the base of the brain, which produces many important hormones including FSH and LH.

placenta (afterbirth): the structure on the wall of the pregnant uterus in which the mother's bloodstream is brought into close proximity with that in the umbilical cord of the fetus, permitting the transfer of nutrients and oxygen to and waste products and carbon dioxide from the growing fetus.

platelets: tiny particles circulating in the blood which are important in the early stages of thrombosis.

progesterone: the other main sex hormone produced by the ovaries (see *oestrogen*). This hormone is produced only in the second half of the menstrual cycle, by the corpus luteum. It prepares the body, especially the uterus, for pregnancy. It is one of the general class of *progestogens*. (A number of artificial progestogens are used along with an artificial oestrogen to produce the combined pill. Their names are given in Tables 9 and 10, pages 186–7, 188.)

progestogen-dominant pill: a combined pill whose biological effects on the body are due more to the relatively higher dose of progestogen it contains than to the oestrogen.

prolactin: a hormone produced by the pituitary gland which stimulates the breasts to produce milk and is also involved in the menstrual cycle.

prostaglandins: natural substances manufactured and released within many tissues of the body. There are many different types with varying effects. Some natural prostaglandins cause the uterus to contract, and these and other artificial variants can therefore be used to cause an induced abortion.

puberty: the time when a boy or girl begins to develop secondary sex characteristics. In a girl, the most important event is the onset of periods, correctly called the menarche.

pyridoxine: this is another name for Vitamin B_6. It is important in body chemistry, particularly relating to the amines which have important functions in the brain.

RH (releasing hormone): there are in fact several releasing hormones, which travel down the stalk of the pituitary gland from the base of the brain, and cause it to release various hormones of its own into the bloodstream. In this book RH has been used to refer to the particular releasing hormone which makes the pituitary release LH and FSH.

spermicide: a substance which is capable of killing sperm. Recommended for contraception when used with another method such as the sheath or the cap, rather than used alone.

sterilization: an operation in a person of either sex which permanently prevents pregnancy, and which is either impossible or difficult to reverse. The definition therefore includes removal of the uterus, or of both ovaries or testicles, though these are only done when necessary because of some disease. More usually, sterilization is achieved by blocking a woman's uterine tubes or a man's vas deferens on each side.

subarachnoid haemorrhage: this is serious bleeding from a

localized weakness of the wall of an artery in the brain, leading to blood appearing in the cerebro-spinal fluid which bathes the brain and spinal cord. It can be fatal or cause prolonged loss of consciousness, but recovery is possible, sometimes with the aid of surgery.

termination of pregnancy: see *abortion.*

testicle (testis): the sex gland of the male in which spermatozoa (sperm) develop, and which also manufactures male sex hormones, especially testosterone.

thrombosis: the formation of a blood clot within a blood-vessel (artery or vein).

uterine (Fallopian) tubes: the tubes which in the female convey the egg to the uterus, and in which fertilization by a sperm usually occurs.

uterus (womb): the hollow organ in women, like other mammals, in which the young develop during pregnancy.

vagina: the distensible passageway which extends from the cervix to the vulva, into which the penis is inserted during intercourse, and which also forms the main part of the birth canal during delivery of a baby.

vas deferens: the tube in the male which conveys the sperm from the epididymis to the base of the penis. It is the tube that is divided at *vasectomy.*

vulva: the name given to the female external genital structures.

100 woman-years: a measure of the frequency of an occurrence in this field. For example, a pregnancy rate of one per 100 woman-years for a given method means that one pregnancy can be expected among 100 women using it for one year (page 47).

Further reading

These and related titles are obtainable from Healthwise, the
FPA Book Shop, Family Planning Association, 27–35 Mortimer
Street, London W1N 7RJ, *Tel.* 071–636 7866, *Fax.* 071–436
3288 (full book list available)—or through a local bookshop if
preferred. They should also be in most public libraries.

All titles are available in paperback editions unless otherwise
stated. All are understandable by lay people, but * beside the
first author signifies a book written primarily for doctors and
students in the field. The date given is the latest edition or
revision.

A. Birth control—the methods

Bromwich, P. and Parsons, A. *Contraception: The Facts*,
   Oxford University Press, 1990
   Updated edition covering all currently available methods of
   contraception. FPA approved.
Flynn, A. and Brooks, M. *A Manual of Natural Family
   Planning*, Unwin Hyman, 1990
   All the most advanced techniques for assessing fertile and
   non-fertile phases in the cycle in order to avoid or plan a
   possible pregnancy. FPA approved.
*Guillebaud, J. *Contraception—Your Questions Answered*,
   Churchill Livingstone, 1989 (revised reprint)
   Comprehensive account of all the reversible methods, readily
   understandable by the general reader. FPA approved.
*Kleinman, R. L. *Family Planning Handbook for Doctors*,
   International Planned Parenthood Federation (IPPF), 1988
   A global but practical perspective: for anyone wanting a
   useful medical account of the available methods.
Mosse, J. and Heaton, J. *The Fertility and Contraception Book*,
   Faber, 1990

Very comprehensive, the pros and cons of each method. With advice to the ordinary reader on how to decide the best method at each stage of life.

* Potts, M. and Diggory, P. *Textbook of Contraceptive Practice*, Cambridge University Press, 1983
Presents a global, medical, view of all aspects of family planning, but emphasizing the common problems encountered in the West.

* Sapire, E. Revised and adapted by Belfield, T. and Guillebaud, J. *Contraception and Sexuality in Health and Disease*, McGraw-Hill, 1990
Contraception is presented within a wider framework of men's and women's reproduction and sexuality, in health and disease.

B. Induced abortion

Gardner, R. *Abortion—the Personal Dilemma*, The Paternoster Press, 1972
A unique, comprehensive account by a Christian gynaecologist of the medical, social, ethical, and spiritual issues of abortion.

* Potts, M., Diggory, P., and Peel, J. *Abortion*, Cambridge University Press, 1977
A fascinating account of historical, sociological, clinical, and population aspects of abortion, worldwide.

Stirrat, G. M. 'Legalized Abortion—the Continuing Dilemma', Christian Medical Fellowship, 1979
Cheap but valuable booklet by a Christian gynaecologist, writing seven years after Gardner (see above).

C. Sexually transmitted diseases (STDs)

* Adler, M. W. *ABC of Sexually Transmitted Diseases*, BMJ, 1990
Articles from the *British Medical Journal* covering diagnosis and treatment, understandable by the general reader. Full colour photographs.

Collier, C. *The 20th Century Plague*, Lion Publishing, 1987
A Christian perspective on the AIDS problem.

Llewellyn-Jones, D. *Sexually Transmitted Diseases*, Faber, 1990
Clear information and advice to potential and actual patients
on the recognition and treatment of the whole range of STDs.

D. Sex and relationships

Delvin, D. *The Book of Love*, New English Library, 1983
Physical and emotional aspects of sex and marriage are
explored together with helpful discussion of the problems.
Rayner, C. *Safe Sex*, Sphere Books, 1987
Small, powerful, and packed with clear, no-nonsense infor-
mation.
Schaeffer, E. *What is a Family?*, Hodder and Stoughton, 1975
A personal view from one woman's experience.
Skynner, R. and Cleese, J. *Families and How to Survive Them*,
Mandarin, 1984
This book shows how understanding gained through family
therapy can lead to happy relationships.
Trobisch, W. *I Married You*, Inter-Varsity Press, 1972
An unusual, extremely readable book on marriage. Based on
the author's experience in Africa, but relevant anywhere.

E. Specially for women

Coope, J. *The Menopause*, Optima, 1988
Cooper, W. *No Change*, Arrow, 1990
Two books which give good reasons why hormone replace-
ment therapy is a good deal, for most women.
Faulder, C. *The Women's Cancer Book*, Virago, 1989
Comprehensive, honest, and reassuring. Cancer is often
preventable and in some cases can be cured.
Kilmartin, A. *Understanding Cystitis*, Arrow Books, 1989
Fully updated guide for sufferers from urinary and related
problems, including thrush. Discusses the causes and treat-
ments, both self-help and medical. With case histories.
Lanson, L. *From Woman to Woman*, Penguin, 1990
Questions and answers about how a woman's body works and
about gynaecological treatments.
Llewellyn-Jones, D. *Everywoman*, Faber, 1989

A gynaecological guide for life, from puberty to the menopause.

Phillips, A. and Rakusen, J. *The New Our Bodies, Ourselves*, Penguin, 1989
A mammoth paperback health book by and for women. British edition of the original version by the Boston Women's Health Book Collective.

Singer, A. and Szarewski, A. *Cervical Smear Test: What Every Woman Should Know*, Optima, 1988
Fully explains the test and what a positive result can mean with detailed descriptions of the treatments. FPA approved.

F. History of birth control

Leathard, A. *The Fight for Family Planning*, Macmillan, 1980
The history of the birth control movement in Britain from 1921: an uphill battle for recognition, culminating in 1974 in the agreement that family planning services should be provided within the National Health Service. Hardback.

G. World population, the environment, and related issues

Schumacher, E. F. *Small is Beautiful*, Sphere Books, 1974
A study of economics as if people mattered.

Taylor, J. *Enough is Enough*, SCM Press, 1975
A book by the Bishop of Winchester, condemning excess of all kinds and in favour of a simpler and more—not less—fulfilling life-style.

Ward, B. and Dubos, R. *Only One Earth*, Penguin, 1972
Concerning the care and maintenance of a small planet.

H. Miscellaneous

* Christopher, E. *Sexuality and Birth Control in Community Work*, Tavistock, 1987
Information of value to anyone but especially the community worker about sexuality, contraception, abortion, and sexually transmitted diseases: the problems presented in different cultures and how to cope with them.

Djerassi, C. *The Politics of Contraception*, W. H. Freeman, 1981
Birth control in the year 2001—critical issues and strategies for the future.
Pauncefort, Z. *Choices in Contraception*, Pan, 1984
Choices, for men and for women.
Smith, M. and Kane, P. *The Pill off Prescription*, Birth Control Trust, 1975
Reasons for widening the range of those empowered to dispense oral contraceptives.
Szarewski, A. *Hormonal Contraception: A Woman's Guide*, Optima, 1991.
As it says in the title; and written by a colleague at the Margaret Pyke Centre.

Useful addresses

This list relates only to the British Isles and cannot be comprehensive. Only a few representative organizations are mentioned and details may have changed since this book went to press. If you have any difficulty, contact a similar organization, ask at your local Town Hall or Citizens' Advice Bureau, or telephone the Family Planning Association (FPA) (see below).

A. Birth control—and related matters

1. *Brook Advisory Centres*
   (Head Office)
   153A East Street
   London SE17 2SD   *Tel.* 071–708 1234

Centres providing a full service in birth control and related matters for young, usually unmarried people, without fuss and without fee.

2. *Family Planning Information Service*
   Family Planning Association
   27–35 Mortimer Street
   London W1N 7RJ   *Tel.* 071–636 7866

Perhaps the most useful address and telephone number of all. Provides free and confidential advice about all methods of birth control, and about sexual problems, clinics for sexually transmitted diseases (STDs), and pregnancy testing. If you have an unplanned or unwanted pregnancy, it can help you to contact the organization of your choice for counselling and help— whether about abortion, adoption, or keeping the baby. Can also inform about other organizations, in this list and others not mentioned. A wide range of *free* leaflets and invaluable FACT SHEETS is available, about all aspects of sexuality.

3. *Irish Family Planning Association*
   Cathal Brugha Street Clinic
   Dublin 1   *Tel.* Dublin (0001) 727276 or 727363

Provides a similar service to the British FPA, but has to charge fees (according to how much you earn) and has to operate within the requirements of Irish law.

4. *Local Family Planning Clinics*

Addresses and opening times best obtained by looking under Family Planning in the telephone book (Business Section) or Yellow Pages of your area. Otherwise contact 2 or 3 above.

5. *Margaret Pyke Centre for Study and Training in Family Planning*
   15 Bateman's Buildings
   Soho Square
   London W1V 5TW   *Tel.* 071–734 9351

The largest centre in Europe for free help with all aspects of birth control and fertility or subfertility. Also houses the population charity known as the Margaret Pyke Memorial Trust.

B. Counselling and more general advice

6. *British Association for Counselling*
   37a Sheep Street
   Rugby
   Warwickshire CV21 3BX   *Tel.* Rugby (0788) 578328

Provides an up-to-date list of local centres that can give expert help on problems concerning sex, drugs, accommodation, and many other matters.

7a. *Chelsea Pastoral Foundation* (for young people aged 18–24)
   155a Kings Road
   London SW3 5TX   *Tel.* 071–351 0839

7b. *Westminster Pastoral Foundation* (all ages)
   23 Kensington Square
   London W8 5HN   *Tel.* 071–937 6956

A full range of counselling services, including individual, marital, and family counselling, Young Person and Serious

Illness counselling services. Cares for people in trouble, uses qualified counsellors from different professional backgrounds.

8. *Lifeline: Pregnancy Counselling and Care*
c/o Rose Cottage
Hillside
Prestatyn
Clwyd LL1 99EN   *Tel.* (0745) 854647

Counselling about unexpected or problem pregnancy: information about the options, help in deciding what to do. Practical and if possible local assistance; and if appropriate, post-abortion counselling.

9. *Rape Crisis Centre*
PO Box 69
London WC1X 9NJ   *Tel.* 071–837 1600 or 071–278 3956

Sympathetic and comprehensive advice about legal, medical, or any other matters, with moral support, for women who have been raped or sexually assaulted.

10. *Relate (formerly National Marriage Guidance Council)*
(Head Office)
Herbert Gray College
Little Church Street
Rugby
Warwickshire CV21 3AP   *Tel.* Rugby (0788) 573241

Has many local branches which run clinics for sexual, relationship, and marriage problems. Details from telephone directory or above.

11. *Salvation Army Counselling Service*
18 Thanet Street
London WC1 9QL   *Tel.* 071–383 4822

Counselling from a Christian basis without any strings or moralizing. Can also inform about help available locally if you live outside London. Also counselling in marital sexual dysfunction.

12. *The Samaritans*
(*London*)
46 Marshall Street
London W1V 1LR   *Tel.* 071–439 2224

Branches in most towns to help the lonely, despairing, or suicidal. Local numbers in the telephone directory.

C. Health

13. *Action on Smoking and Health (ASH)*
    5–11 Mortimer Street
    London W1N 7RH   *Tel*. 071–637 9843
Everything to help the prospective ex-smoker.

14. *Health Education Authority*
    Hamilton House
    Mabledon Place
    London WC1H 9TX   *Tel*. 071–383 3833
Information and free leaflets and posters on all aspects of how to stay healthy.

15. *Sexually Transmitted Diseases*
    Special Clinics
Local clinics are usually listed in the telephone directory under VD or Venereal Diseases or as above. Otherwise ask Casualty Department of local hospital or contact FPA (A2 above).

16. *Women's Health Concern*
    Alexandra House
    Oldham Terrace
    London W3 6NH   *Tel*. 071–938 3932
Practical help with women's health problems, especially those related to the menstrual cycle and the menopause.

17. *Women's Health and Reproductive Rights*
    Information Centre (WHRRIC)
    52–4 Featherstone Street
    London EC1 8RT   *Tel*. 071–251 6580
The title describes what is on offer.

18. *Women's National Cancer Control Campaign*
    Suna House
    128 Curtain Road
    London EC2 3AR   *Tel*. 071–729 4688
Information and free leaflets on all aspects related to cancer in women.

D. People in special categories

Support groups for those with long-term illnesses of all kinds (such as diabetes, endometriosis, multiple sclerosis, etc.): The King's Fund, 126 Albert Street, London NW1 7NF (*Tel.* 071–267 6111) should be able to help by supplying addresses and contacts.

19. *SPOD (The Association to Aid Sexual and Personal Relationships of People with a Disability)*
    286 Camden Road
    London N7 0BJ   *Tel.* 071–607 8851

Help in a previously much-neglected area for people with any relevant disability.

E. Birth and babies, single parents

20. *Gingerbread*
    35 Wellington Street
    London WC2E 7BN   *Tel.* 071–240 0953

A self-help group for one-parent families, with 350 branches.

21. *Maternity Alliance*
    15 Britannia Street
    London WC1X 9JP   *Tel.* 071–837 1273

Advises about getting fit for pregnancy. Send s.a.e. for invaluable leaflets.

22. *National Childbirth Trust*
    Alexandra House
    Oldham Terrace
    London W3 6NH   *Tel.* 081–992 8637

Everything to help expectant mothers and fathers during pregnancy, childbirth, and breast-feeding. Issues leaflets and booklist, and address list for local classes (fees charged).

23. *National Council for One-Parent Families*
    255 Kentish Town Road
    London NW5 2LX   *Tel.* 071–267 1361

Offers advice without strings or pressures, and in confidence. Acts as a link between self-help groups like number 20, local social workers, and others providing services for single pregnant girls and single mothers or fathers.

F. World population, the environment, and related issues

A few of many organizations which might be mentioned. See page 17 for further details about their work.

24. *The Conservation Trust*
    George Palmer Site
    Northumberland Avenue
    Reading RG2 7PW   *Tel.* (0734) 868442

25. *Friends of the Earth*
    377 City Road
    London EC1V 1NA   *Tel.* 071–837 0731

26. *International Planned Parenthood Federation*
    Regent's College
    Inner Circle
    Regent's Park
    London NW1 4NS   *Tel.* 071–486 0741
(This links together the individual Family Planning Associations of the world.)

27. *Marie Stopes International*
    129 Whitfield Street
    London W1P 5RT   *Tel.* 071–388 3034

28. *Population Concern*
    231 Tottenham Court Road
    London W1P 9AE   *Tel.* 071–631 1546 or 071–637 9582

29. *Tear Fund (The Evangelical Alliance Relief Fund)*
    11 Station Road
    Teddington
    Middlesex TW11 8QE   *Tel.* 081–977 9144

30. *World Wide Fund for Nature*
    Panda House
    Weyside Park
    Godalming
    Surrey GU7 1XR   *Tel.* 0483–426444

World directory of pill names

Only pills containing 50 mcg of oestrogen or less are listed, and all so-called 'sequential' pills are omitted. This directory is based on the *Directory of Hormonal Contraceptives* compiled by Ronald Kleinman and published by the International Planned Parenthood Federation, 1988. The groups by letter A to E are those used in Table 9 (pages 186–7), Table 10 (page 188), Table 12 (page 221), and Figure 17 (pages 190–1), so that a pill brand identified here can be fitted into the scheme described in Chapters 7 and 8.

Caution: Occasionally, the same or a very similar name is used in different parts of the world for quite different formulations (e.g. Noriday). So recheck the stated formulation of a pill in the list here against that of any previously used packets which you are attempting to match, and discuss the matter with a doctor or pharmacist. He or she can also tell you if a 28-day (Every Day) version is available, if not mentioned here (see pages 52, 61).

Abbreviations

Oestrogens		ethinyloestradiol	EE
		mestranol	MEE
Progestogens	Group A	norgestimate	NGM
	Group B	gestodene	GSD
	Group C	desogestrel	DSG
	Group D	levonorgestrel	LNG
	Group E	norethisterone (in N. America called norethindrone)	NET
Also relatives of NET		norethisterone acetate	NEA
		ethynodiol diacetate	EDDA
		lynestrenol	LYN

NB Many other brands exist worldwide, but only those which are identical or very similar to UK brands are listed here. Those available in Britain are in *italics*.

⁺ means that the pill also contains (non-contraceptive) dextronorgestrel.

Group A (Norgestimate, NGM)

Micrograms	*Micrograms*	
EE 35 +	NGM 250	*Cilest.*

Group B (Gestodene, GSD)

Micrograms	*Micrograms*	
EE 30 +	GSD 75	*Femodene, Femodene ED*, Femodeen, *Minulet*, Femovan, Ginoden, Gynera, Gynovin, Minulet, Minulette, Myvlar.

Group C (Desogestrel, DSG)

Micrograms	*Micrograms*	
EE 30 +	DSG 150	Desolett, Frilavon, *Marvelon*, Marviol, Microdiol, Planum, Practil, Prevenon, Varnoline.
EE 20 +	DSG 150	*Mercilon*, Myralon.

Group D (Levonorgestrel, LNG)

Micrograms	*Micrograms*	
EE 50 +	LNG 250	Anfertil, Anulit,⁺ Contraceptive HD, Denoval, D-Norginor, Duoluton, Duotone, Euginon,⁺ Eugynon 0.25, Eugynon,⁺ Eugynon 50,⁺ Eugynona,⁺ Evanor,⁺ Evanor-d, Femenal,⁺ Follinett, Follinyl,⁺ Gentrol,⁺ Gravistat, Gravistat 250, Mithuri,⁺ Mithuri Red,⁺ Monovar, Neogentrol, Neo-Gentrol 250/50, Neogynon, Neogynona, Neo-Primovlar, Neovlar, Noral, Nordiol, Norginor, Normanor, Novogyn, Novogynon, Ovadon, Ovidon, Ovlar, Ovoplex, Ovral,⁺ Ovral 0.25, *Ovran*, Pil KB, Planovar,⁺ Primovlar,⁺ Primovlar 50, Stediril,⁺ Stediril-d.

EE 50 +	LNG 125	Ediwal, Gravistat 125, Microgynon, Microgynon 50, Minigynon 50, Minules, Neo-Gentrol 125/50, Neo-Stediril, Nordet 50, Regunon, Stediril 50.
EE 30 +	LNG 250	Combination 5, *Eugynon 30*, Nordiol 30, *Ovran 30*, Primovlar 30.[+]
EE 30 +	LNG 150	Ciclo, Contraceptive LD, Egogyn, Follimin, Gynatrol, Levlen, Lo-Femenal,[+] Lo-Gentrol,[+] Lo-Ovral,[+] Lo/Ovral,[+] Microginon, Microgyn, *Microgynon 30*, Microvlar, Minidril, Minigynon 30, Minivlar, Min-Ovral,[+] Mithuri Green,[+] Neo-Gentrol 150/30, Neomonovar, Neovletta, Nordet, Nordette 150/30, Ovoplex 30/150, Ovoplexin, Ovral L,[+] Ovranet, *Ovranette*, Rigevidon, Stediril-d 150/30, Stediril-M, Suginor.

Triphasic formula

EE 30 +	LNG 50	
EE 40 +	LNG 75	Fironetta, *Logynon*, *Logynon ED*,
EE 30 +	LNG 125	Triagynon, Triciclor, Trigynon, Trikvilar, Tri-Levlen, *Trinordiol*, Trionetta, Triphasil, Triquilar, Triquilar ED, Trisiston, Triviclor.

Group E (Norethisterone, NET)

Micrograms	*Micrograms*	
EE 50 +	NET 1000	Alovan, Anovulatorio MK, Arona, Non-Ovlon, Norlesterire, Ovcon 50.
MEE 50 +	NET 1000	Anogenil, Combiginor, Conceplan, Conlumin, Floril, Genora 1+50, Gulaf, Maya, Mithuri Blue, Nor-50, Norethin 1/50, NorFor, Noriday, Noriday 1+50, Norimin, Norinyl, *Norinyl-1*, Norinyl-1/28, Norinyl 1/50, Norinyl 1+50, Norit, Novulon 1/50, Orthonett, Orthonett 1/50, Ortho-Novin, *Ortho-Novin 1/50*, Ortho-Novum, Ortho-Novum 1/50, Ortho-Novum 1+50, Perle, Plan mite, Regovar, Regovar 50, Ultra-Novulane.

EE 35 +	NET 1000	Brevicon-1+35, Brevinor-1, Genora 1+35, Gynex 1/35E, Nelova 1+35E, Neocon, *Neocon 1/35*, Neo-Norinyl, Norethin 1/35, *Norimin*, Norinyl 1+35, Norquest-Fe, Ortho 1+35, Ortho-Novum 1+35, Ortho-Novum 1/35, Ovysmen, Ovysmen 1/35.
EE 35 +	NET 500	Brevicon, *Brevinor*, Conceplan mite, Gynex 0.5/35E, Micro Plan, Moda Con, Modacon, Modicon, Nelova 0.5/35E, Neo-Ovopausine, Nilocon, Norminest-Fe, Orthonett-Novum, Ovacon, *Ovysmen*, Ovysmen 0.5/35, Perle LD.

Biphasic formulae

EE 35 +	NET 500	⎫
EE 35 +	NET 1000	⎬

Binovum, Ortho 10/11, Ortho-Novum 10/11 (second two are equivalent to *Binovum*, page 187, but give 3 extra days at the lower dose).

Triphasic formulae

EE 35 +	NET 500	⎫
EE 35 +	NET 750	⎬
EE 35 +	NET 1000	⎭

Ortho 777, Ortho-Novum 777, Triella, *TriNovum*, *TriNovum ED*. See page 187.

EE 35 +	NET 500	⎫
EE 35 +	NET 1000	⎬
EE 35 +	NET 500	⎭

Synfase, Synfasic, *Synphase*, Synphasec, Synphasic, Tri-Norinyl. See page 187.

Group E continued (Norethisterone acetate, NEA)

Micrograms	*Micrograms*	
EE 50 +	NEA 1000	Anovlar, Anovlar 1 mg, Anovulatorio, Berligest, Celapil, Estrinor, Gynophase, Logest 1/50, Milli-Anovlar, Minovlar, Minovlar ED, Nodiol, Non-Ovlon, Norit, Norlestrin 1 mg, Norlestrin 1/50, Norlestrin Fe 1 mg, Orlest, Orlest 21, Orlest 1 mg, Prolestrin, Rosanil, Zorane 1/50.
EE 30 +	NEA 1500	*Loestrin 30*, Loestrin 1.5/30, Loestrin Fe 1.5/30, Logest 1.5/30, Minestril-30, Zorane 1.5/30.

| EE 30 + | NEA 1000 | Econ 30, Econ mite, Milli-Anovlar, Trentovlane. |
| EE 20 + | NEA 1000 | Loestrin, *Loestrin 20*, Loestrin 1/20, Loestrin Fe 1/20, Lostrin 1/20, Minestril-20, Minestrin 1/20, Nogest, Zorane 1/20. |

Group E continued (Ethynodiol diacetate, EDDA)

| *Micrograms* | *Micrograms* | |
| EE 30 + | EDDA 2000 | Conova, *Conova 30*, Demulen 30. |

Group E continued (Lynestrenol, LYN)

| *Micrograms* | *Micrograms* | |
| EE 37.5 + | LYN 750 | Ginotex, Lyndiol 0.75, Micro-Ovostat, Minilyndiol, Minipregnon, Ministat, Ovamezzo, Ovoresta M, Ovoresta micro, Ovostat-Micro, Pregnon, Restovar. |

Phasic pills: as in Table 9 (pages 186–7), for comparison with the monophasics the *average daily* doses given in the British brands are shown below:

	Micrograms	*Micrograms*
Logynon/Trinordiol	EE 32.4 +	LNG 92
Binovum	EE 35 +	NET 833
TriNovum	EE 35 +	NET 750
Synphase	EE 35 +	NET 714

Continuous progestogen-only pills (POPs)

	Micrograms	
Group A	NGM	not yet available.
Group B	GSD	not yet available.
Group C	DSG	not yet available.
Group D	LNG 37.5	*Neogest,*[+] Ovrette,[+] Postinor.
	LNG 30	Follistrel, Microlut, Microluton, *Microval*, Mikro-30, Mikro-30 Wyeth, *Norgeston*.
Group E	NET 35	Conceplan-Micro, Dianor, Micronett, *Micronor*, Micro-Novum, Micronovum, *Noriday*, Noriday-1, Noridei, Nor-QD.

	NET 30	Conludag, Gesta Plan, Mini-Pe, Minipill.
Group E continued	EDDA 0.5	Continuin, *Femulen*.
Group F	LYN 0.5	Exlutena, Exluton, Exlutona, Minette.

Index

For names of pills, see World directory of pill names (page 301) and Chapters 7, 8. Appendices (pages 261 onwards) are not indexed. See Glossary (page 283) for definitions of technical terms.

abdomen, pain in, 75, 218; *see also* cramps
abortion, 14, 23, 80, 165; not contraception, 169–70, 234–6, 239; starting pill after, 57, 210
abstinence, 29, 59, 82
acne, 71, 136, 154, 158, 160, 168, 204
age
    and heart attacks, 98; and POP, 209, 221; and smoking and the pill, 104–7, 149–50, 166
AIDS and HIV, 2, 26–8, 225, 234, 252
albumin, 88
allergic rhinitis, 115
allergy/immunity system, 89, 115, 136, 137–8, 157, 183; allergy to pill itself, 137, 177; *see also* immune methods of contraception
amenorrhoea, 127, 181; *see also* periods; hormone withdrawal bleeds
amines, 108, 111
ampicillin, 70
anaemia, 91, 147, 157, 158, 159, 179
androgenic effects, 204, 244
angina, 173
antibiotics, 70–1, 214; *see also* drugs
antibodies, 137, 237–9, 247
anti-coagulants, 76, 95
anti-thrombin III, 88, 93
arterial diseases, 96–102, 154–6, 173; and smoking, 98, 99, 100, 105–7
arthritis, 133, 137, 138
asthma, 115
atherosclerosis, *see* arterial diseases
atrial fibrillation, 173
auto-immune disorders, 137

baby, breast-fed, effect of pill hormones on, 170, 222–3, 240, 257
baby, unborn, effect of pill hormones on, 127–30, 176, 215
bacteria, 71, 118, 120
barrier methods, 59, 252–3, 254, 257; *see also* cap; sheath
benign intracranial pressure (BICP), 114
bile disorders, 116, 117, 175
bilharzia, 148
binding globulins, 89, 91
biphasic pills, 186–7, 192–6
birth defects, 127–30
birth rate statistics, world, 12–18
bladder infections, 117–18
bleeding
    abnormal vaginal, 176, 199–200; after ending of early pregnancy, 57; causing strokes, 100, 102–3, 171; menstrual, *see* periods; on combined pill, *see* hormone withdrawal bleeds; on POP, *see* periods on POP; *see also* breakthrough bleeding; haemorrhage
blood clotting
    disorders, 87, 88, 93–9, 101, 171, 173; risk during immobilization or surgery, 76, 171, 174; tests, 148, 154, 178; *see also specific types of thrombosis*
blood diseases, 173
blood fats (lipids), 87, 88, 90, 97, 152–3, 154–6, 172, 188, 189, 217; diseases involving, 88, 90, 96–7, 99, 172; tests, 154–6, 178

blood groups, 95, 98
blood platelet aggregation, 88, 93
blood pressure, 100, 102–3, 153;
checks on, 75, 80, 82, 84, 100, 103;
effect of combined pill on, 89,
102–3, 150, 153, 154, 155, 161, 172,
179, 185, 197; effect of POP on,
217, 221, 222; past or family history of raised, 102, 172, 177, 179
blood sugar, *see* glucose
body chemistry, 86–93, 149, 151,
152–6, 189, 192, 217
body water, *see* fluid retention
bones and joints, 133
bowel thrombosis, 101
brain
as hormone controller, 32; *see also*
pituitary gland; side-effects of pill
on, 108–14; *see also specific types
of brain disease*
breaks from pill-taking, 76, 149–51;
between pill packets, effectiveness
during, 53–4, 60–62, 71
breakthrough bleeding, 55, 59, 65–6,
72, 73, 155, 192–4, 199–201; and
epilepsy, 113; when taking other
drugs, 72, 73, 113, 183, 199
breast-feeding, 49; and the pill, 57,
170; and the POP, 222–3, 210, 240;
contraceptive effect of, 18, 240
breasts
cancer, 132, 138–42, 175, 184;
check at family planning visit, 81;
benign disease, 132, 139, 142, 156,
158, 160, 184; enlargement,
131, 203; milky discharge, 88,
132–3; self-examination procedure,
81, 139, 185; tenderness and
tingling, 74, 132, 184, 203, 194, 218
breathlessness, 75
bursitis, 137

calf pain, 75, 94, 96; *see also* deep
venous thrombosis
cancer
and the pill, 138–46, 151–52; and
smoking, 50–1, 107; past history
of, 175; *see also* breasts; cervix;
ovaries; uterus; vagina

candida infection, 119–20
cap, 2, 21, 59, 61, 68–9, 104, 181,
234, 253, 255, 257–9
carpal tunnel syndrome, 75, 136
CASH Study, 143, 144
central nervous system, 108–14
cerebral haemorrhage, 100
cerebral thrombosis, 99–100; *see also*
strokes
cervix, 33, 46; cancer of, 28, 107,
138, 184; cervical ectopy (erosion),
119, 201; cervical mucus, 46, 49,
120, 208, 209, 210, 229; cervical
smear test, 28, 81, 84, 138, 184,
185; trans-cervical sterilization, 237
chest pain, 75
chicken pox, 137
chilblains, 137
Chinese Medical Journal, 245
chlamydia, 25, 120, 218
chloasma, 134, 157, 161, 222
cholesterol, *see* blood fats
chorea, 113, 176
choriocarcinoma, 144
cilia, 27, 34
circulatory disorders, 85–107, 149–57,
153–6; family history of, 172, 178;
past history of, 171–3
clotting factors, 87, 88, 93, 94, 148, 152
coil, *see* IUD
combined pill
compared with other methods,
251–4; contra-indications, 171–84,
219–20; duration of use, effect of,
104, 127, 149–52, 180; history,
42–4; how it works, 38, 46, 47–51;
ideal scheme for safe use, 184–5,
196–204; past use, possible effects
of, 126–8, 149–52; rules for starting
to take, 54–7, 79, 193; *see also
specific diseases*; side-effects of
combined pill; Chapters 2–7, 10
conception, 8, 37, 41; after coming
off pill, 77, 126–8, 149, 181; after
the POP, 216–17
condom, *see* sheath
cone biopsy, 184
connective tissue diseases, 173
contact lenses, 114,

contraception
 future new methods, 229–49;
  history, 8–11; ideal method, 226–7;
  present choices, 250–9; proportion
  using various methods in UK,
  20–2; *see also specific methods*
contraceptive vaginal ring, 224–5
contra-indications
 to combined pill, 171–84, 219; to
  POP, 219–20
coronary thrombosis, *see* heart
 disease
corpus luteum, 33, 35, 37, 40, 41, 42,
  43, 50; and other contraceptive
  methods, 235, 238; *see also* luteal
  phase; luteinizing hormone
counselling, 1, 30–1, 79, 80–1, 82, 83,
  84, 110–11, 198, 200–1, 205
cramps
 menstrual, 42, 124, 160, 197; as
  affecting legs, 74, 136
Crohn's disease, 116, 137
cystitis, 117–18
cysts, ovarian, 122, 160, 218, 219

D & C, 57, 144, 222
deafness, 176
deep venous thrombosis, 57, 76,
  94–5, 149, 161, 168, 171
Depo-Provera (DMPA), 174, 229,
  232, 251, 180, 240, 255–6
depression, 108–10, 182, 206, 222;
  anti-depressive drugs and pill, 182
desogestrel, 90, 155, 186, 189, 191,
  192
developing countries, 12–18, 91; risks
  of pill in, 147–8
diabetes, 87, 95, 97, 98, 155, 172,
  178, 221
Dianette (cyproterone acetate pill),
  204
diaphragm, 253, 254, 255, 257; *see
  also* cap
diarrhoea, 67; on POP, 211, 214
diet, 91, 92, 99, 128, 147, 148; and
  migraine, 111
diethylstilboestrol (DES), 129
Dioscorea plant, 11
diosgenin, 11, 43

dizziness, 136, 203, 204, 205, 218
drug interaction, 58, 67, 70–2, 182–3,
  199, 214, 220–1
drug regulatory committees
 (including FDA, CSM), 44, 105,
  141, 150
drugs for male contraception, 243–8
dummy pills, 52, 195, 204
duodenal ulcers, 115–16
dysmenorrhoea, 49, 124, 160

ectopic pregnancy, 79, 121, 218–19,
  251, 252, 257
eczema, 135–7
egg, fertilization of, *see* fertilization
egg-release, 32–8, 39–40, 77, 78, 79,
  233; effect of POP on, 208, 211;
  nasal spray preventing, 232–3;
  occurring while on pill, 57, 59,
  62–72; pill's prevention of, 42, 45–6;
  see also Mittelschmerz; ovaries
egg sacs, *see* follicles
embolism, 94
embryo, 37, 41, 238
emergency contraception, 64, 78–9,
  212, 214, 234
endometriosis, 122, 203
endometrium, 33, 45, 50, 119, 122,
  124, 143–4
epilepsy, 70, 71, 75, 112–13, 182–3,
  214
epiphyses, 133
erythema multiforme, 135, 177
erythema nodosum, 135
ethinyloestradiol, 43, 91–2, 102, 153,
  154, 186–7, 189, 204
ethynodiol diacetate, 186–7, 188, 221
Every Day (28-day) packaging, 52,
  62, 193, 195
eye trouble, 75, 101, 102, 114

failure of pill, 47, 155, 182, 183, 194,
  201, 202; failure of POP, 209, 210,
  212–13, 214–15; *see also* missing
  tablets
fainting, 75; *see also* dizziness
Fallopian tubes, *see* uterine tubes
Family Planning Association (FPA),
  22, 55, 104, 105, 168

family planning clinics, 79–81, 184
family planning methods, *see*
  contraception
Femring, *see* contraceptive vaginal
  ring
fertility, 8–11, 126–7, 181; *see also*
  conception after coming off pill
fertilization, 8, 37, 229, 231; and
  contraception, 10, 235–6, 239,
  240–1
fibrinolysis, 88, 93
fibroids, 121–2, 156
fimbriac, 33, 35
fingers, excessive whitening of, 136
fluid retention, 89, 92–3, 182, 203
folic acid, 89, 91, 128
follicles, 32, 33, 34, 35, 38–9, 40, 42,
  46, 62, 123, 125
follicle stimulating hormone (FSH),
  33, 34, 38, 39, 40, 41, 42, 123; and
  combined pill, 38, 42, 45, 46, 88;
  and POP, 208; and menopause,
  221; and analogues of releasing
  hormone (RH), 232–3
follicular phase, 36, 39–40
forgetting tablets, *see* missing tablets
FSH, *see* follicle stimulating hormone

gall-bladder, 116, 117, 159, 161, 175
gallstones, 76, 117, 154, 175
gastric flu, 137
German measles, 82–3
gingivitis, 136
glucose (blood sugar), 87, 88, 90, 155
Glucose Tolerance Test, 87, 179, 217
gonorrhoea, 24, 25
gossypol, 245–6
gums, inflammation of, 136

hCG, *see* human chorionic
  gonadotrophin
HDL$_2$-cholesterol, 154–5, 193
haemorrhage
  intracerebral, 100; subarachnoid,
  100; *see also* bleeding
hair problems, 135, 136, 204
hands, whitening and 'deadness', 136
hay fever, 115, 137
headaches, 52, 74, 75, 101, 112, 149,
  205, 218, 222; *see also* migraine
heart disease, 90, 92, 97, 97–8, 105,
  147, 149–51, 155–6, 159, 161, 171,
  173, 178, 219
hepatitis, 24, 175
herpes gestationis, 135, 176
herpes virus, 25, 28
hirsutism, 135, 136, 204
Hodgkin's disease, 183
hormone pregnancy tests, 129
hormones, changes in body's own,
  88, 90, 91; *see also specific
  hormones*
hormone withdrawal bleeds, 38,
  47–9, 52, 63, 65–6, 73, 86, 124–5,
  127, 192, 194–5; absence of 49, 53,
  66, 73, 125, 127, 183, 201, 202;
  postponement of, 53, 124–5,
  194–5; *see also* breakthrough
  bleeding; periods on POP
human chorionic gonadotrophin
  (hCG), 37, 41, 129, 144–5, 176,
  235, 238
hypercholesterolaemia, 90
hyperlipidaemia, 90
hypertension, 102–3; *see also* blood
  pressure; pulmonary hypertension
hypothalamus, 32, 33, 45
hysterectomy, 121, 175, 258

immobilization and thrombosis, 76,
  95, 171, 174, 220
immune methods of contraception,
  237–9, 248
immunity/allergy system, *see*
  allergy/immunity system
implantation, 37, 41, 46, 78, 233,
  234, 235, 236
infectious disease, 137
infertility, natural, 239–40
inhibin, 245
injectable contraceptives, 174, 229,
  232, 240, 251, 255–6
insulin, 87, 88, 90, 155, 217, 221; *see
  also* diabetes
internal (vaginal) examination, 81–2,
  84, 122, 219
intestinal disorders, 115–17
intracerebral haemorrhage, 100

intra-cervical devices, 233
intra-uterine devices, *see* IUD
irritability, *see* 'nerves'
itching, 25, 117, 119; *see also* rashes
IUD (intra-uterine devices), 2, 21, 22, 78, 79, 104, 183, 218, 233, 234, 236, 237, 258, 259

jaundice, 75, 88, 116–17; of pregnancy, 117, 175, 176
joints and bones, 133

kidney disease, 92, 102, 172, 182

leg aches and cramps, 74, 75, 136; thrombosis in superficial veins, 154, 161; *see also* deep venous thrombosis; varicose veins
leprosy, 148
leukaemia, 173
levonorgestrel, 154–5, 186–7, 188, 190, 221, 222
LII, *see* luteinizing hormone
libido, 74, 110, 159, 204, 218, 243
lipids, *see* blood fats
liver, 67, 70, 116–17, 145, 148, 175; fluke infection, 148; and male pill, 244; thrombosis affecting, 102; tumours of, 145
long-term effects of pill, 104, 138, 149–52, 180
loop, *see* IUD
lower dose of pill, changing to, 72–3, 193
luteal phase, 35–6, 41–2
luteinizing hormone (LH), 33, 34, 35, 38, 39, 40, 41, 42, 45, 46; and combined pill, 38, 42, 45; and POP, 208; and other contraceptive methods, 233, 241, 244–6
lynestrenol, 188

major surgery, 76, 174, 220
malaria, 148
male contraceptive methods, 241–8, 252, 254
male pill, 11, 20, 242–6
mass media, 168–9, 249
medicines, *see* drugs

melanoma, 145
melasma, *see* chloasma
menopause, 139, 221, 258, 259
menorrhagia, 121, 124
menstrual cycle, 32–42, 123–5, 133; good effects of combined pill on, 38, 47–9, 123–6, 160; reversibility of effects on cycle, 149, 162; *see also* hormone withdrawal bleeds; modified on POP, 207–8, 214–16, 217–18; *see also* periods; pill cycle
mesenteric thrombosis, 101
mestranol, 43, 188
migraine, 75, 100–1, 111–12, 171–2, 177, 180, 185
minerals, effect of pill on body's, 89, 91
mini-pill, *see* progestogen-only pill (POP)
miscarriage, 57, 80, 129, 210, 236
missing tablets, 47, 57, 58–65; on POP, 211–14
Mittelschmerz, 40, 124, 125
monilial infection, *see* candida infection
'morning after' methods, *see* emergency contraception
mucus, *see* cervical mucus
mucus method of contraception, 59, 240
multiple sclerosis, 183
myasthenia gravis, 183

nasal spray contraceptives, 232–3
natural family planning (safe period), 8–9, 21, 22, 59, 240–1, 254
nausea, 50, 74, 147, 203, 222; and POP, 215, 222; and underweight, 115, 197
'nerves' and irritability, 182, 203, 205; *see also* depression
neural tube defects (NTDs), 127–8
neurodermatitis, 135
norethisterone, or its acetate, 43, 154, 155, 187, 188, 191, 221
norethynodrel, 43
Noristerat, 229
Norplant, 232
numbness, 75

nurses, 17, 80, 84

obesity, *see* overweight
oestradiol, 42
oestrogen, 33–46, 47, 60, 62, 70, 71,
  88, 208; in the pill, 1, 38, 42–6,
  101, 136, 137, 181, 197, 203, 204;
  in ultra-low-dose pill, 153–4, 185,
  186–7, 196; conditions affected by
  (according to dose in pill), 93–6,
  153–4, 197, 203, 204; effect on
  epiphyses, 133; and emergency
  contraception, 78, 234
oestrogen-dominant pills, 194, 203–4
'once-a-month' contraception, 235
operations and thrombosis, 76, 95,
  174–5, 220
Oral Contraception Study (RCGP),
  see Royal College of General
  Practitioners' Study
orgasm, female, 8
osteoporosis, 133–4
otosclerosis, 176
ovaries, 32–42, 43, 45, 47, 48, 49, 50,
  123, 158; and POP, 218, 219–20;
  cancer, 50, 138, 144, 146, 152, 158;
  cysts, 123, 158, 218, 219–20
overdose of pill, 85–6
overweight, risk of thrombosis, 94,
  95, 96, 98, 99, 172; special
  supervision on pill, 180, 181; *see
  also* weight gain
ovulation method, *see* natural family
  planning
ovulation pain, *see* Mittelschmerz
ovulation process, *see* egg-release
Oxford/FPA Study, 104, 105, 108,
  116, 118, 121, 126, 129, 137, 142,
  146, 147, 165, 182, 218

papilloedema, 114
pelvic infection, 25, 120, 156, 233,
  251, 252, 257
penis, 24, 25, 228, 230, 242, 248
periods, normal menstrual, 36, 37,
  42, 124; absence of, 32, 49–50,
  76–7, 126–7, 181, 217; pain during,
  42, 124, 158, 160; return of, after
  coming off pill, 76–7, 126–7, 181,

197, 217
'periods' on combined pill, *see*
  hormone withdrawal bleeds
periods on POP, 207, 214, 215,
  217–18
phasic pills, 50, 53, 64, 124, 125, 155,
  186–7, 192–5, 200–1, 202
phlebitis, *see* superficial veins
phlegm, blood-stained, 75
photosensitivity, 134
pill cycle, 48
pill-free interval/week, 47–9, 53–4,
  62, 63, 64, 65, 73, 113, 151, 182
pill ladders, 189, 190–1, 195, 204
pill usage statistics, 20–2
pill Victims Action Group, vii
pituitary gland, 32–42; and the pill,
  38, 41, 46, 62; disorder, 131, 182;
  adenoma, 131; and male
  contraception, 244–5
plant products, 10–11, 43
platelet, aggregation, 88, 93, 94
poisoning, absence of pill effect, 85–6
polyarteritis nodosa, 173
polycythaemia, 173
polyps, uterine, 176, 201
POP, *see* progestogen-only pill
population problem, 11–18
porphyrias, 134, 176
post-coital contraception, *see*
  emergency contraception
post-natal blues, 110; *see also*
  depression
postponement of periods, 49, 53,
  124–5, 194–5
pregnancy
  bleeding after end of early, 57; and
  German measles, 82–3; how it
  happens, 32–41; mimicked by pill,
  49–50, 74, 86, 93, 176; pill-taking
  during early, 66, 78–9, 129–30,
  176; and POP, 215, 216, 218;
  reduced protection by combined
  pill, 58–72; reduced protection by
  POP, 211–14; risks during, 86, 93,
  95, 165–6; starting pills after, 55–7;
  starting POP after, 210; becoming
  pregnant after coming off pill,
  76–7, 126–7, 127–30; *see also*

ectopic pregnancy

pregnancy tests, 61, 66, 69, 83, 129, 202; after coming off pill, 77, 130; while on POP, 213, 215

pre-menstrual tension, 19, 125, 160, 194

prescription, pill off, 17

progesterone, 33, 34, 36, 37, 38, 41, 42, 88, 234, 235, 238, 241; *see also* progestogens

progestogen-dominant pills, 120, 121, 132, 153–6, 203–4

progestogen-only pill (POP), 2, 145, 156, 174, 205–6, 207–23, 251, 257, 258; and age, 221–2; and breast-feeding, 57, 170, 222–3; changing from combined pill to, 211; changing to combined pill from, 211 ; contra-indications, 219–20; effect on periods, 214–15, 217–18, 221–2; and FSH, 208, 221; health risk, 156, 217–19, 220–22; interactions with other drugs, 214; method of action 207–9, 215–16, 236; missing tablets, 211–14, 215; nausea with, 215, 222; and ovaries, 218, 219; and pituitary gland, 216; and pregnancy, 214, 215; rules for starting, 210; side-effects less than with combined pill, 103, 111, 112, 156, 217–19, 222; and smoking, 221; when to take, 209–10

progestogens, 42; in combined pill, 1, 42, 118, 136, 137, 153–6, 181, 186–92, 196, 197, 202–4; conditions worsened or improved by (according to dose in pill), 118, 120, 122, 132, 153–6, 197, 202–4; in POP, 221, 222–3; in other contraceptive methods, 229, 232–3, 234; lipid-friendly (selective), 90, 155–6, 181, 189, 192, 199, 217, 220

prolactin, 42, 88, 131, 182

prostaglandins, 42, 124, 235

publicity, 3, 4, 20, 168–9, 249

Puerto Rican pill trials, 44, 51

pulmonary embolism, 94–5

pulmonary hypertension, 173

pyridoxine, 89, 108, 110

rashes, 26, 75, 137; *see also* allergy/immunity system

Raynaud's syndrome, 136

releasing hormone (RH), 33, 39, 42, 232, 245

reliability of pill research, 147

respiratory disorders, 115, 137

retinal thrombosis/bleeding, 102

RH, *see* releasing hormone

rheumatoid arthritis, 133, 137

rhythm method, *see* natural family planning

riboflavine, 89

risk, excess or attributable, due to pill, 103–7, 163, 164–7

risks and benefits, of combined pill, 3–5, 6, 157–70; of POP, 217–23

rosacea, 135

Rotor syndrome, 175

Royal College of General Practitioners' (RCGP) Study, 103–5, 106, 109, 112, 115, 118, 121, 129, 135, 136, 137, 147, 149, 150, 155, 158, 160–1, 165, 167, 179, 205

RU 486, 234, 235

Rubella, 81–2

rule for overall safety of pill method, 87

rules if contraceptive action reduced combined pill, 58–72; POP, 211–15

'safe' period (rhythm method), *see* natural family planning

saliva tests, for contraception, 241; for safety of pill, 152

sarcoidosis, 183

screening tests, 152

sedatives, 70

sex education, 257

sex drive, *see* libido

sexually transmitted diseases (STDs), 23–8, 80, 120

sexual responsibility, 23–7, 28–31; *see also* counselling; under-age sex

sheath, 2, 20, 21, 22, 23, 27, 54, 59, 61, 66, 67, 68–9, 71, 78, 79, 128, 165, 181, 210, 211, 212–13, 248, 252, 254, 257, 259

sickle cell anaemia, 179–80, 251

side-effects of combined pill, 4, 5, 49–51, 73–6, 85–156, 157–62; beneficial, 49–51, 158, 160, 163, 168; absolute contra-indications, 171–7; relative contra-indications, 177–84; list of potentially serious symptoms, 75; pill ladders to minimize, 189–204; summary of side-effects, 157–61

side-effects of POP, 217–19; contra-indications to POP, 219–20

skin disorders, 134–6, 137, 145, 160–1, 222

smoking, 50–1, 70, 80, 164; and age, 105–6, 150–1, 163; and arterial diseases, 88, 93–100, 105–6; and bronchitis, gangrene, cancer, and death risks, 106; and circulatory diseases, 88, 93–100, 104–6, 150, 151, 172, 180; and heart attacks, 97–9; and migraine, 111; and POP, 221; and strokes, 100; and venous thrombosis, 95; and Vitamin C, 92

sores and warts, 25

speech disturbances, 75, 101

sperm, 8, 37, 41, 46, 208, 228, 229, 230–1, 233, 234, 237, 239, 240–1, 243, 244–8, 254;

spermicides, 9, 59, 233, 247, 250, 252, 253, 254, 255, 259

sponges for contraception, 234, 250, 254, 257

spotting, see breakthrough bleeding

STDs, see sexually transmitted diseases

sterilization (female), 20, 21, 22, 76, 174, 178, 236–7, 253–4, 257, 258

stomach upsets while on pill, 66–9; while on POP, 211–13

strokes, 90, 99–100, 101, 102, 149–51, 154, 159, 161, 171–2

subarachnoid haemorrhage, 100

sulphasalazine, 245

sunlight sensitivity, 134

superficial veins, thrombosis in, 96, 154, 161, 171

symptothermal method, 240; see also natural family planning

synovitis, 137

syphilis, 24, 25

systemic lupus crythematosus (SLE), 137, 173

teenagers and the pill, 133, 139, 140, 181; see also under-age sex

telangiectasia, 135

temperature method, including new variants, 41, 59, 240, 254; see also natural family planning

tenosynovitis, 137

termination, see abortion

testosterone, 244–5

thrombosis, 88–9, 93–101; during immobilization or operation, 75, 94, 95, 171, 174; during pregnancy, 86, 93, 95, family history of, 178; past history of, 171; see also specific types of thrombosis

thrush, 119

thyroid disease, 90–1, 138

thyroid gland hormones, 42, 88, 90

tooth extraction, dry socket after, 136

toxaemia of pregnancy, 98, 179

toxicity of pill, 85–6

toxic-shock syndrome, 120–1

tranquillizers, 70

transaminases, 88

trichomonas vaginitis (TV), 120

'tricycle' system, 52–3, 111, 113, 183

triphasic pills, see phasic pills

trophoblastic disease, 144–5, 176

tropical diseases, 147–8

tuberculosis, 70, 71, 182–3

twin pregnancies after pill-use, 128; during pill-use, 129

ultrasound scanning, 241

under-age sex, 82, 133

underweight, 115, 148, 197

urethritis, 25

urinary infections, 117–18, 137, 161

urine tests, 80, 117, 152, 241; see also pregnancy tests

urticaria, 134

uterine (Fallopian) tube, 33, 34, 35, 37, 40, 41, 46, 208, 218; and

sterilization, 236–7, 253–4, 257; *see also* ectopic pregnancy
uterus, 33, 35–7, 40–2; cancer of (equals cancer of endometrium), 138, 143–4, 146, 152, 158, 175; irregular bleeding from, 57, 176, 199–201, 217, 221–2; pill's effect on lining of, 37, 41–2, 46, 47–9, 192, 208; *see also* endometrium, hysterectomy

vagina
cancer of, 130; discharge and the pill, 74, 82, 118–19, 203; discharge and STDs, 24, 25, 120; dryness, 110, 118, 204; examination (internal), 81–2, 84; infections, 24, 119–20; pessaries and sponges, 232, 234, 250
variable dose pill, *see* phasic pills
variation in blood levels of pill hormones, 197–9
varicose veins, 95–6, 180–1
vasectomy, 20, 21, 22, 243, 247–8, 254, 257, 258
veins, thrombosis in, 94–6, 101–2, 149, 154, 171; and smoking, 95; *see also* blood clotting; deep venous thrombosis; superficial veins, thrombosis in
venereal disease (VD), *see* sexually transmitted diseases (STDs)
vertigo, 136
vision disturbances, 75, 101, 102, 114; *see also* eye trouble
vitamins, 89, 91–2, 108–9, 110, 111, 128, 148
vitamin C, 91–2
voice changes in singers linked with pill, 136
vomiting while on pill, 66–9, 197; on POP, 211–14

Walnut Creek Study, 104, 105, 137, 147, 165
wart virus, 25, 28
wax in ears, 136
weight checks, 80, 84
weight gain, 74, 92–3, 149, 218, 222; *see also* fluid retention; overweight; underweight
withdrawal method, 248, 254
womb, *see* uterus
women's role in society, 18–20
World Fertility Survey, 16
World Health Organization (WHO), 11, 91, 103, 128, 130, 148, 229, 235, 246

yam roots, 11, 43

zona pellucida, 239

Acknowledgements

Illustrations by Illustra Design Limited, Susan Walker, and the Technical Graphics department of OUP.

OXFORD

MORE OXFORD PAPERBACKS

Details of a selection of other Oxford Paperbacks follow. A complete list of Oxford Paperbacks, including The World's Classics, Twentieth-Century Classics, OPUS, Past Masters, Oxford Authors, Oxford Shakespeare, and Oxford Paperback Reference, is available in the UK from the General Publicity Department, Oxford University Press (RS), Walton Street, Oxford, OX2 6DP.

In the USA, complete lists are available from the Paperbacks Marketing Manager, Oxford University Press, 200 Madison Avenue, New York, NY 10016.

Oxford Paperbacks are available from all good bookshops. In case of difficulty, customers in the UK can order direct from Oxford University Press Bookshop, 116 High Street, Oxford, Freepost, OX1 4BR, enclosing full payment. Please add 10 per cent of the published price for postage and packing.

MEDICINE IN OXFORD PAPERBACKS

Oxford Paperbacks offers an increasing list of medical studies and reference books of interest to the specialist and general reader alike, including The Facts series, authoritative and practical guides to a wide range of common diseases and conditions.

CONCISE MEDICAL DICTIONARY
Third Edition

Written without the use of unnecessary technical jargon, this illustrated medical dictionary will be welcomed as a home reference, as well as an indispensible aid for all those working in the medical profession.

Nearly 10,000 important terms and concepts are explained, including all the major medical and surgical specialities, such as gynaecology and obstetrics, paediatrics, dermatology, neurology, cardiology, and tropical medicine. This third edition contains much new material on prenatal diagnosis, infertility treatment, nuclear medicine, community health, and immunology. Terms relating to advances in molecular biology and genetic engineering have been added, and recently developed drugs in clinical use are included. A feature of the dictionary is its unusually full coverage of the fields of community health, psychology, and psychiatry.

Each entry contains a straightforward definition, followed by a more detailed description, while an extensive cross-reference system provides the reader with a comprehensive view of a particular subject.

Also in Oxford Paperbacks:

Drugs and Medicine   Roderick Cawson and Roy Spector
Travellers' Health: How to Stay Healthy Abroad 2/e
Richard Dawood
I'm a Health Freak Too!
Aidan Macfarlane and Ann McPherson
Problem Drinking   Nick Heather and Ian Robertson

SCIENCE IN OXFORD PAPERBACKS

Oxford Paperbacks' expanding science and mathematics list offers a range of books across the scientific spectrum by men and women at the forefront of their fields, including Richard Dawkins, Martin Gardner, James Lovelock, Raymond Smullyan, and Nobel Prize winners Peter Medawar and Gerald Edelman.

THE SELFISH GENE
Second Edition
Richard Dawkins

Our genes made us. We animals exist for their preservation and are nothing more than their throwaway survival machines. The world of the selfish gene is one of savage competition, ruthless exploitation, and deceit. But what of the acts of apparent altruism found in nature—the bees who commit suicide when they sting to protect the hive, or the birds who risk their lives to warn the flock of an approaching hawk? Do they contravene the fundamental law of gene selfishness? By no means: Dawkins shows that the selfish gene is also the subtle gene. And he holds out the hope that our species—alone on earth—has the power to rebel against the designs of the selfish gene. This book is a call to arms. It is both manual and manifesto, and it grips like a thriller.

The Selfish Gene, Richard Dawkins's brilliant first book and still his most famous, is an international bestseller in thirteen languages. For this greatly expanded edition, endnotes have been added, giving fascinating reflections on the original text, and there are two major new chapters.

'learned, witty, and very well written . . . exhilaratingly good.' Sir Peter Medawar, *Spectator*

'Who should read this book? Everyone interested in the universe and their place in it.' Jeffrey R. Baylis, *Animal Behaviour*

'the sort of popular science writing that makes the reader feel like a genius' *New York Times*

Also in Oxford Paperbacks:

The Extended Phenotype Richard Dawkins
The Ages of Gaia James Lovelock
The Unheeded Cry Bernard E. Rollin

WOMEN'S STUDIES FROM
OXFORD PAPERBACKS

Ranging from the *A–Z of Women's Health* to *Wayward Women: A Guide to Women Travellers*, Oxford Paperbacks cover a wide variety of social, medical, historical, and literary topics of particular interest to women.

DESTINED TO BE WIVES
The Sisters of Beatrice Webb

Barbara Caine

Drawing on their letters and diaries, Barbara Caine's fascinating account of the lives of Beatrice Webb and her sisters, the Potters, presents a vivid picture of the extraordinary conflicts and tragedies taking place behind the respectable façade which has traditionally characterized Victorian and Edwardian family life.

The tensions and pressures of family life, particularly for women; the suicide of one sister; the death of another, probably as a result of taking cocaine after a family breakdown; the shock felt by the older sisters at the promiscuity of their younger sister after the death of her husband are all vividly recounted. In all the crises they faced, the sisters formed the main network of support for each other, recognizing that the 'sisterhood' provided the only security in a society which made women subordinate to men, socially, legally, and economically.

Other women's studies titles:

A–Z of Women's Health   Derek Llewellyn-Jones
'Victorian Sex Goddess': Lady Colin Campbell and the Sensational Divorce Case of 1886   G. H. Fleming
Wayward Women: A Guide to Women Travellers
Jane Robinson
Catherine the Great: Life and Legend   John T. Alexander

THE WORLD'S CLASSICS

A 250–strong series of the finest editions of the greatest works of world literature from Homer to Hardy.

'Must now be the most wide-ranging and well-chosen list of its kind.' *London Evening Standard*

ARMADALE

Wilkie Collins

Edited with an Introduction by Catherine Peters

'it has the immense—and nowadays more and more rare—merit of never being dull'

T. S. Eliot's appreciation of *Armadale* still stands. The third of Wilkie Collins's four great novels of the 1860s, coming after *The Woman in White* and *No Name*, and immediately before *The Moonstone* (all available in World's Classics), *Armadale* is quintessentially a novel of its decade. It deals with the emergence of the autonomous, sexually active woman from the dichotomies of Madonna and Magdalen; with the legal tangles of the unsatisfactory marriage laws; with the perception of the growing role of scientific intrusion into the privacy of the individual psyche. Above all, it explores the divided self, and the need to acknowledge the darker side of the personality: a modern theme grafted on to a traditional melodrama, and worked out with all Collins's skill in handling a complex and exciting plot.

First published in 1866, the text of this World's Classics edition is that of the one-volume 1869 edition, checked and corrected against both the first impression and the magazine serialization which preceded it.

Also available in the World's Classics:

Nicholas Nickleby Charles Dickens
A Hazard of New Fortunes William Dean Howells
Middlemarch George Eliot
Melmoth the Wanderer Charles Maturin

CLASSIC ENGLISH SHORT STORIES

The four volumes of *Classic English Short Stories* have been compiled to reflect the excellence and variety of short fiction written in English during the twentieth century. Each volume covers a different period and represents the most distinguished writers of their day.

THE DRAGON'S HEAD

This collection contains stories written in the years between the turn of the century and the outbreak of the Second World War—'a restless and impatient age'. The authors include John Galsworthy, 'Saki', Naomi Mitchison, H. G. Wells, Dorothy L. Sayers, and Somerset Maugham.

THE KILLING BOTTLE

This collection brings together 12 very different authors whose short stories, written in the 1940s and 1950s, helped establish or extend their reputations as writers of stories, novels, or poetry. The 12 include Evelyn Waugh, Elizabeth Bowen, Graham Greene, V. S. Pritchett, Dylan Thomas, and Frank O'Connor.

CHARMED LIVES

This collection contains stories written in the 1950s and 1960s, many of which demonstrate the impressive and accomplished skills of Commonwealth writers who began to achieve world-wide reputations during that period, including Ruth Prawer Jhabvala, Nadine Gordimer, H. E. Bates, Bill Naughton, L. P. Hartley, and Peter Ustinov.

THE GREEN MAN REVISITED

This collection includes works written in the 1960s and 1970s by authors living all around the world, including Chinua Achebe, Kingsley Amis, Susan Hill, Olivia Manning, V. S. Naipaul, William Trevor, John Updike, and Patrick White.

A SPLENDID QUARTET OF SHORT STORIES

CLASSIC IRISH SHORT STORIES
Selected and Introduced by Frank O'Connor

The Irish short story, Frank O'Connor believes, is 'a distinct art form' and the stories he has chosen for this collection show how the form has remained peculiarly itself while being developed in various ways in response to changing social and political conditions. Authors include James Joyce, Liam O'Flaherty, Seàn O'Faolàin, George Moore, and Elizabeth Bowen.

CLASSIC ENGLISH SHORT STORIES
Selected and Introduced by Derek Hudson

The years 1930 to 1955 marked a high point in the fortunes of the English short story. Inevitably the Second World War left its mark on many of the tales Derek Hudson has collected here, but, he argues, the dominating impression is that very English characteristic, humour. The authors include Somerset Maugham, Virginia Woolf, Evelyn Waugh, Graham Greene, H. E. Bates, and Rosamond Lehmann.

CLASSIC SCOTTISH SHORT STORIES
Selected and Introduced by J. M. Reid

CLASSIC AMERICAN SHORT STORIES
Selected and Introduced by Douglas Grant

Also in Oxford Paperbacks:

CLASSIC ENGLISH SHORT STORIES

The Dragon's Head
The Killing Bottle
Charmed Lives
The Green Man Revisited

OXFORD BOOKS

Oxford Books began in 1900 with Sir Arthur Quiller-Couch ('Q')'s *Oxford Book of English Verse*. Since then over 60 superb anthologies of poetry, prose, and songs have appeared in a series that has a very special place in British publishing.

THE OXFORD BOOK OF ENGLISH GHOST STORIES

Chosen by Michael Cox and R. A. Gilbert

This anthology includes some of the best and most frightening ghost stories ever written, including M. R. James's 'Oh Whistle, and I'll Come to You, My Lad', 'The Monkey's Paw' by W. W. Jacobs, and H. G. Wells's 'The Red Room'. The important contribution of women writers to the genre is represented by stories such as Amelia Edwards's 'The Phantom Coach', Edith Wharton's 'Mr Jones', and Elizabeth Bowen's 'Hand in Glove'.

As the editors stress in their informative introduction, a good ghost story, though it may raise many profound questions about life and death, entertains as much as it unsettles us, and the best writers are careful to satisfy what Virginia Woolf called 'the strange human craving for the pleasure of feeling afraid'. This anthology, the first to present the full range of classic English ghost fiction, similarly combines a serious literary purpose with the plain intention of arousing pleasing fear at the doings of the dead.

'an excellent cross-section of familiar and unfamiliar stories and guaranteed to delight' *New Statesman*

Also in Oxford Paperbacks:

The Oxford Book of Short Stories   edited by V. S. Pritchett
The Oxford Book of Political Anecdotes
edited by Paul Johnson
The Oxford Book of Ages
edited by Anthony and Sally Sampson
The Oxford Book of Dreams   edited by Stephen Brock